From Nursing Homes to Home Care

From Nursing Homes to Home Care

Marie E. Cowart, DrPH
Jill Quadagno, PhD
Editors

Routledge
Taylor & Francis Group
LONDON AND NEW YORK

First published 1996 by The Haworth Press, Inc.

Published 2013 by Routledge
711 Third Avenue, New York, NY 10017, USA
2 Park Square, Milton Park, Abingdon, Oxfordshire OX14 4RN

First issued in paperback 2016

Routledge is an imprint of the Taylor & Francis Group, an informa business

From Nursing Homes to Home Care has also been published as *Journal of Aging & Social Policy,* Volume 7, Numbers 3/4 1996.

Library of Congress Cataloging-in-Publication Data

From nursing homes to home care/Marie E. Cowart, Jill Quadagno, editors,
p. cm.
Includes bibliographical references and index.
ISBN 978-1-315-82524-3 (eISBN)
ISBN 978-1-56024-826-2 (alk. paper)
1. Aged-Long-term care-United States. 2. Aged-Long-term care-Govemment policy-United States. I. Cowart, Marie E. II. Quadagno, Jill S.

HV1461.F75 1996 96-14870
362.6-dc20 CIP

ISBN 13: 978-1-138-97477-7 (pbk)
ISBN 13: 978-1-56024-826-2 (hbk)

From Nursing Homes to Home Care

CONTENTS

ABOUT THE EDITORS

Marie E. Cowart, DrPH, is Research Associate at the Pepper Institute on Aging and Public Policy and Professor of Health Systems Planning in the Department of Urban and Regional Planning at Florida State University in Tallahassee. In addition to a number of positions she holds for the development and implementation of health policy in Florida, Dr. Cowart conducts research on health and long term care policy concerns. Her most recent article publications have appeared in the *Journal of Applied Gerontology, AIDS and Public Policy Journal,* and *Nursing Economics.* She is the co-editor of *Nurses in the Workplace,* which was published in 1992.

Jill Quadagno, PhD, is Professor of Sociology at Florida State University in Tallahassee, where she holds the Mildred and Claude Pepper Eminent Scholar's Chair in Social Gerontology. The former Vice-President of the American Sociological Association, she recently served as Senior Policy Analyst on the President's Bi-Partisan Commission on Entitlement and Tax Reform. Professor Quadagno has conducted extensive research on Florida's Medicaid System and is the author or editor of seven books, among which are *The Transformation of Old Age Security; States, Labor Markets and the Future of Old Age Policy;* and, most recently, *The Color of Welfare: How Racism Undermined the War on Poverty.*

Foreword: Health Care Reform, Long-Term Care, and the Future of an Aging Society

On September 22, 1993, President Clinton unveiled his health care reform plan before a Joint Session of Congress. At that time, the Administration held a "Health Care University," in which, for the first time in congressional history, the Administration held seminars for members of Congress to explain and answer their questions on the Health Security Act. One of the Act's centerpieces was the President's long-term care proposal. In its simplest form, the proposal would provide, for the first time, a national system of home and community-based care that would be based not on age, but on levels of disability called Activities of Daily Living (ADLs). It would give states tremendous flexibility to use the allocated money to provide a full array of home and community-based long-term care, including important social services such as transportation, meals, and vouchers.

A year after the President came before Congress, it was apparent that the outcome of any health care reform in that session was unlikely, despite negotiations attempting to establish some kind of health care reform. The crisis still exists, and the reason for having attempted to establish universal health and long-term care remains. None of the problems that brought us to that point have changed. If anything, they have worsened. We stand to benefit, however, from the tremendous debate and struggle that occurred during the first year.

There is a silver lining to the struggle during the first year–the issue of long-term care. In the first half of the year, Congress was saying that, whatever might happen to health care reform, long-term care was a non-

---

[Haworth co-indexing entry note]: "Foreword: Health Care Reform, Long-Term Care, and the Future of an Aging Society." Torres-Gil, Fernando M. Co-published simultaneously in *Journal of Aging & Social Policy* (The Haworth Press, Inc.) Vol. 7, No. 3/4, 1996, pp. xiii-xviii; and: *From Nursing Homes to Home Care* (ed: Marie E. Cowart and Jill Quadagno) The Haworth Press, Inc., 1996, pp. xiii-xviii. Single or multiple copies of this article are available from The Haworth Document Delivery Service [1-800-342-9678, 9:00 a.m. - 5:00 p.m. (EST)].

starter; it was dead. It was too expensive. The Congress was not hearing from constituents that long-term care was what they wanted. The Administration on Aging (AoA) was told that it could assume long-term care and prescription drugs were out in any final or later negotiations, as the Congress went into their deliberations. After hearing that, the Administration on Aging consulted with constituency and advocacy groups. Many appointees were called to testify before various congressional committees, before "supportive" members who believed deeply in long-term care.

The result is that the original long-term care proposal has remained in every one of the legislative proposals under debate, and has remained essentially in its original form. The issue of long-term care, then, is on the top of the political, congressional, and public agendas. This was reinforced in President Clinton's proposed 1995 Budget Resolution to eliminate the deficit. His proposal included an investment in long-term care by reintroducing his earlier home and community-based long-term care program—an investment critically needed even as we seek to address the deficit problem. Long-term care is here to stay, and therefore it is our job to continue the momentum into the years ahead.

In addition, we must recognize that long-term care, however addressed, must include the issues of aging and disability. Aging, disability, and long-term care policy are inexorably linked, and we no longer have the luxury of keeping these three issues separate. We can no longer think of long-term care solely as an aging issue, or as programs for older persons, much less nursing homes, as opposed to home and community-based care; rather, we must look at long-term care as a vehicle for all ages, young and old. In fact, the nation's demographics are compelling us to move in that direction.

I have a personal interest in this topic. I contracted polio when I was very young and I have lived with a lifelong disability. Thanks to many people, and Shriner's Hospital, I have adapted and have grown older with this disability. As I and my baby-boomer colleagues reach our middle ages, I realize more and more that issues of, and services for, older persons are as relevant to me as they are to a younger person with a disability. There are tremendous benefits to be gained from a partnership between the disability community, aging advocates, and those who are supporting and promoting long-term care.

The 1990 census shows that persons 65 and older now account for 12% of our population, or roughly 32 million people. More than half of them are disabled. Even more interesting is that two thirds are in minority groups. This compares with a disability rate for the population as a whole of just under 20%. By the year 2030, one in five Americans will be 65 or older, compared with one in eight today. Some think those figures are relatively conservative. As society ages, as the first of the baby-boom generation reaches retirement age in the next decade, and as younger persons with disabilities become older, we must begin to plan ahead to prepare for their aging and to address the issues of aging, disability, and long-term care.

However, the issues of long-term care, aging, and disability are not just about the demographics. They are important issues for women who are, by and large, the caregivers of our families and communities. They are important issues for families who increasingly are finding that addressing long-term care for any of their family members is a great financial pressure, as well as an emotional and physical responsibility. This is compelling, because it is about reinventing government. It's about using limited resources and finding common needs for services rather than affording separate delivery systems. Although there is a window of opportunity in this decade to begin to address that issue and plan for the aging of the baby boomers, that window will begin to close relatively quickly. We may only have this decade to plan somewhat rationally for what will be twice as many older persons and many more persons with disabilities in the years ahead.

The position of Assistant Secretary for Aging was created recently to give aging a broader context throughout the Administration. It strengthens the ability of the Department of Health and Human Services (HHS), of AoA, and of aging advocates to address this issue in a cross-cutting manner. Responsibility can no longer be delegated to one agency, discipline, or cabinet department. It involves everyone. That includes the Administration on Aging, the Health Care Financing Administration, the Public Health Service, the Department of Housing and Urban Development, the Department of Transportation, even the Treasury Department. These issues of long-term care transcend our near categories of regulations, legislation, and funding sources.

The Administration has formed a working group on disability. Health and Human Services is addressing the issues of aging, disability, and long-term care in various ways. In particular, the Social Security Administration recently unveiled a plan for a new disability claims process that will make the Disability Insurance system more user-friendly and save millions of dollars in administrative costs in that program over the long run. The Departments of Transportation and HHS have formed a joint coordinating council to insure that transportation is a vital element in any long-term care system. In HHS, there are a number of interagency agreements between the Office of Planning and Evaluation and AoA to conduct a number of critical studies, for example, analyzing board-and-care regulations and their effects on the quality of care. The Administration on Aging also is conducting a national study on assisted living that examines the areas of housing and services for the frail elderly and the disabled, as well as collecting and analyzing more data about the long-term care infrastructure and the services currently provided by the aging network.

Recently, the Administration on Aging and the Administration for Children and Families signed a first-ever interagency agreement that will examine the abuse, neglect, and exploitation of elderly persons in domestic settings and long-term care facilities, including those of our Native American tribal organizations. Another joint partnership has been struck between the Administration and the Health Care Financing Administration. HCFA has traditionally been viewed as the "money bags" because it distributes Medicare and Medicaid funds, and AoA has often been viewed as the "do-good" social service agency that provides important social services, but the two have not collaborated to any significant degree. In the last two years, HCFA and AoA have begun work on joint projects to promote long-term care through the use of Medicaid waivers and by utilizing the aging network's social services. AoA also has supported a number of programs that provide direction in this area, including four national resource centers on long-term care and thirteen demonstration projects that include disability issues. Long-term care and disability, then, are now priorities of not just AoA, but also the Department of Health and Human Services. Other initiatives that HHS and AoA are developing include focusing on older women's issues. The Older Women's Initiative was recently unveiled, which addresses long-term care and women's roles as the caregivers in society. More time and resources will be put into the provision of nutrition programs. Often, one meal a day can mean the difference between a frail person remaining in his or her home and moving into a nursing home. A "blueprint" initiative has been developed to plan ahead for the aging of the baby boomers. Part of the initiative is studying how we can move toward a long-term care policy that prepares us for twice as many retirees in the next century.

These efforts reflect a commitment to the importance of moving toward universal long-term care. There is a recognition that any future expansion of long-term care policy must be predicated on several criteria. First, more resources will be devoted to home and community-based care. Second, states must have flexibility, because each state is unique. Third, whatever is developed must include disabled persons of all ages. Finally, whatever is developed must be based on measures of quality and outcome, not quantity, so that it improves the quality of life for the individual recipient. A consensus is growing among members of Congress and the Administration as well as among many scholars and policy analysts in this area.

Taking this approach, however, won't be easy. First, there are still differences between the aging and disability communities. In part, this is because some disability groups are concerned that the "clout" of seniors might detract from their efforts to gain visibility for their own concerns. As for senior citizen groups, there exist some concerns that if they share services with the younger disabled, it may detract from the types of services provided for older persons.

There is also concern among both groups about how they will share limited resources. The President's long-term care proposal, for example, allocated two thirds of the services to older persons and one third to the younger disabled. However, there are many examples that the program can work and is working. For example, in 1993, the Administration on Aging conducted its first national survey on long-term care programs and services provided by the aging network. It found that the aging network, which is composed of 57 state offices on aging, 670 area agencies on aging, 5,000 senior centers, and thousands of providers, was already heavily engaged in this area. In fact, nine state offices on aging oversee not just aging, but long-term care and programs for younger disabled persons. Nineteen states are already using Medicaid waivers to provide long-term care services to both populations.

However, we do have to take into account some macro or "big-picture" policy concerns. Major debates are taking place in Congress about the nature of entitlement programs. Those include all programs for middle-income groups and big business, such as tax subsidies. Unfortunately, however, some people view entitlement programs solely in terms of Social Security and Medicare. There is discussion about coming up with proposals that might cut Medicare and Social Security programs, "means-test" them, or change their eligibility criteria. Any changes are going to alter the course of those programs.

In addition, in the Department of Health and Human Services, the Social Security Administration became an independent organization in March of 1995. Part of Social Security's domain is disability insurance. The separation leaves one small agency, the Administration for the Developmentally Disabled (ADD), within HHS. The Administration on Aging will work closely with ADD and other areas of the department to provide leadership on disability policy.

The ongoing debates on health care reform have yet to play themselves out. I remain sanguine that the American public will support some type of substantive reform. The public is increasingly realizing that big government is not the problem–that, in fact, it may be insurance companies who control supply and demand and decide who gets services and who doesn't. The public is beginning to realize that the lack of universal long-term care and health care is ultimately affecting everyone. It is still uncertain when this crisis will reach a critical mass. Some said that if nothing were to happen in 1995, there eventually will be even greater pressures for a single-payer type of approach.

Be that as it may, we should not wait for national government or public pressure to force us to act. It is important that state and local providers move forward in building, refining, and expanding their systems in long-term care, because whatever may or may not happen at the federal level, the compelling need to have universal long-term care to address the needs of older persons and those with disabilities is only going to grow. As those entities move forward and make progress, the political and democratic system ultimately will catch up.

Fernando M. Torres-Gil, PhD
Administration on Aging
Washington, DC

From Nursing Homes to Home Care: Introduction

In the United States, long-term care policy for the aged and disabled consists of a fragmented system of care. It is divided between states and the federal government, between several programs (Medicare, Medicaid, and the Older Americans Act), and between the family, the hospital, and the nursing home. The current system of care, which still encourages institutional care rather than home care, is distasteful to older people who would prefer to remain in their own homes. It has also become an increasing burden on states whose coffers are being depleted by the rising costs of Medicaid payments to nursing homes.

The issues involved in reforming our current system are complex, and there is no consensus on the approach to use. But there is no doubt that the need exists, and that need will grow as the baby boomers approach retirement age. In the next decade, we face crucial decisions: how best to blend formal and informal services, how to assure quality of care and quality of life in long-term care policy, how to finance the programs we devise, which health needs to address, and whether to use regulatory or competitive approaches.

In September 1994, we invited some of the nation's most prominent experts on long-term care policy to prepare papers for a conference at Florida State University. The conference papers are presented in this volume. The focus of the papers is on the shift to services provided in the home. All of the authors address the recent trend to home and community-based care, that is, the range of services provided by programs such as Community Care for the Elderly and the Medicaid Waiver programs under section 2176. The exceptions are the paper by Peter Shaughnessy and colleagues, who examine traditional home care services such as those reimbursed by Medicare, and the paper by Vicki Freedman and Peter

---

[Haworth co-indexing entry note]: "From Nursing Homes to Home Care: Introduction." Cowart, Marie E. and Jill Quadagno. Co-published simultaneously in *Journal of Aging & Social Policy* (The Haworth Press, Inc.) Vol. 7, No. 3/4, 1996, pp. 1-2; and: *From Nursing Homes to Home Care* (ed: Marie E. Cowart and Jill Quadagno) The Haworth Press, Inc., 1996, pp. 1-2. Single or multiple copies of this article are available from The Haworth Document Delivery Service [1-800-342-9678, 9:00 a.m. - 5:00 p.m. (EST)].

Kemper, who examine a broader range of formal in-home services in the United States and in other countries.

The objective of these papers is not to formulate a single answer to the questions about long-term care, but to arm educators and policymakers with the information they will need in the coming years to participate knowledgeably in these debates.

We gratefully acknowledge the support of the Mildred and Claude Pepper Foundation in the funding of the conference. We also appreciate the support provided by Jill R. Norton in guiding this project through the editing process.

Marie E. Cowart, DrPH
Jill Quadagno, PhD
Florida State University

POPULATION AGING AND THE RISK OF DISABILITY

Ways of Thinking About the Long-Term Care of the Baby-Boom Cohorts

Eric R. Kingson, PhD

Boston College
Chestnut Hill, Massachusetts

SUMMARY. In examining various ways of thinking about the development of long-term care policy for the baby-boom cohorts, this

---

Eric R. Kingson is Associate Professor, Graduate School of Social Work, Boston College.

The author expresses his appreciation to the Pepper Institute on Aging and to the American Association of Retired Persons for funding and facilitating research upon which this article draws (Eric Kingson, *The Diversity of the Baby Boom Generation: Implications for Their Retirement Years* [Forecasting and Environmental Scanning Department, American Association of Retired Persons, April, 1992]).

Dr. Kingson can be contacted at the Graduate School of Social Work, Boston College, Chestnut Hill, MA 02167.

[Haworth co-indexing entry note]: "Ways of Thinking About the Long-Term Care of the Baby-Boom Cohorts." Kingson, Eric R. Co-published simultaneously in *Journal of Aging & Social Policy* (The Haworth Press, Inc.) Vol. 7, No. 3/4, 1996, pp. 3-23; and: *From Nursing Homes to Home Care* (ed: Marie E. Cowart and Jill Quadagno) The Haworth Press, Inc., 1996, pp. 3-23. Single or multiple copies of this article are available from The Haworth Document Delivery Service [1-800-342-9678, 9:00 a.m. - 5:00 p.m. (EST)].

article discusses the importance of basing long-term care policy discussions on a recognition of social and economic trends, as well as on the informal exchanges of care that occur over life and the diversity within the baby-boom cohorts. The implications of two ways of thinking about challenges posed by the aging of baby boomers–the generational equity/crisis perspective and the generational investment/gradual adjustment perspective–are also discussed. It is suggested that the generational equity perspective is consonant with proposals to expand private savings for long-term care contingencies and private long-term insurance and, secondarily, with proposals to expand means-testing for benefits. The second perspective is more consistent with proposals to create new universal services through a traditional social insurance approach, or through a block grant such as the one discussed in the context of the Clinton health care reform plan. *[Article copies available from The Haworth Document Delivery Service: 1-800-342-9678.]*

As baby boomers in the United States are called upon to assist with the care of their elders and later as they face greater exposure to risks associated with their own functional disabilities, long-term care will assume growing prominence as a public concern. This article examines various ways of thinking about long-term care for baby boomers–the 76 million people born between 1946 and 1964. It begins by discussing trends that need to be taken into consideration. Next, it reviews why long-term care policy discussions need to be based upon recognition of the importance of the informal exchanges of care that occur over people's lifetimes, primarily in the context of the family. The benefits and costs of caregiving transfers become clear in this context, as do issues of particular concern to women. The final section presents two ways of thinking about challenges posed by the aging of baby boomers–the generational equity/crisis perspective and the generational investment/gradual adjustment perspective. The differing implications of each of these views for long-term care policy discussions are then discussed. The article contains much conjecture, which is shared because it is useful to think about different ways that policy issues–some far off and some close at hand–may be structured by the information we consider relevant and the perspectives we apply.

TRENDS AND UNCERTAINTIES

Thinking about long-term care policy for the baby-boom cohorts must recognize (1) population changes and the uncertainties surrounding forecasts, (2) changing dependency ratios, (3) the diversity of the baby-boom cohorts, (4) the growing risk of long-term care, and (5) economic uncertainty.

Population Aging and the Baby Boom: Knowns and Unknowns

Between 1946 and 1964, 76 million people were born in the United States–17 million more individuals than would have been born had the fertility patterns of the early 1940s prevailed. Taking immigration into account, baby boomers numbered roughly 78 million people in 1990, nearly one third of the U.S. population (Lewin-VHI, Inc., 1994). As baby boomers moved from nurseries to schools and then to the employment and housing markets, the size of this "macro cohort" created strains, necessitating adjustments in social institutions. Today, attention is beginning to focus on the implications of millions of baby boomers swelling the ranks of the old.

Anticipated demographic trends. Barring unforeseen calamities, the baby-boom cohorts will age in a society that is older, more populous, and more diverse than previous generations. As a result of birth and mortality trends and the aging of the baby-boom cohorts, the population age 65 and older and, to an even greater extent, the population age 85 and older, are expected to grow very rapidly over the next 60 years–both in absolute numbers and as a percentage of the entire population. Under its middle series projections, the U.S. Bureau of the Census (Day, 1992) estimates that there will be about 54 million people age 65 and older by 2020 (20.2% of the population), and 79 million by 2050 (20.6% of the population) compared to 31 million (12.55%) in 1990. Baby boomers will represent about 60 million of the projected 70 million people aged 65 and older by 2030. Very significantly, given the association between advanced old age and functional disabilities, the Bureau projects that by 2050 almost 18 million people (4.6% of the population)–virtually all baby boomers–will be age 85 and over compared to 3.1 million (1.3%) in 1990.

Starting around 2010, baby boomers will begin a roughly 60-year transition into and eventually through old age, with the oldest cohort reaching age 65 in 2011 and age 85 in 2031, and the youngest 65 in 2029 and 85 in 2049. Beth Soldo and Emily Agree (1988) note that "Because of the staggered impact of [their] aging . . . [c]oncerns about financing retirement will give way to focus on the ability of health care programs to absorb very old and probably frail elders" (p. 14).

Older populations will be more diverse; younger populations, even more so (Day, 1992). By 2035, the various populations considered minorities at risk are projected to constitute more than half of the population under age 20 (Day, 1994), with the white non-Hispanic population[1] declining as a percentage of the total population from 75.7% in 1990, to 67.6% in 2010, and to 52.7% in 2050.

Uncertainties of projections. Forecasts are uncertain, and the "margin for error" is larger for long-term forecasts. Agencies that develop population estimates provide ranges revising estimates as new information becomes available (see Day, 1992). Considerable variation exists in the projected size of the population as a whole, and in the absolute and relative numbers of old (65 and over) and very old persons (85 and over). Some assess that elderly population estimates based on Social Security Administration's (SSA) high cost projections (see Board of Trustees, 1994) and on the Census Bureau's highest series estimates may provide a more realistic basis for charting retirement and health care policy than other series. Most participants in a 1993 workshop convened by the Institute of Medicine to assess survival, health, and disability forecasting placed greater confidence in a model that projected higher life expectancies and larger elderly populations for the long term, 84.3 years at birth in 2050 compared to 82.1 under the Census Bureau's 1992 middle series (Institute of Medicine, 1993).

A question for the future with potentially important public policy implications is whether the anticipated increases in life expectancy at older ages will be matched by parallel reductions in morbidity and disability as the baby-boom cohorts age. A substantial literature addresses this question but is not conclusive (Verbrugge, 1991). Findings from recent research (Manton, Cordor, & Stallard, 1993), however, seem to point increasingly to an aggregate decrease in disability among older populations, especially among more highly educated and high-income older persons.

Changing Dependency Ratios

Changing old-age support ratios, commonly termed "old-age dependency ratios," enters into most discussions of the implications of population aging. As the number and proportion of older persons change during the next 60 years, the number of persons aged 18 through 64, the so-called working-age population, is projected to decline as a proportion of the entire population. The ratio of elderly persons (65 and older) to every 100 "working age" persons has increased from about 15:100 persons in 1955 to roughly 21:100 today, and is expected to increase to about 36:100 persons in 2030, when all surviving baby boomers are 65 or older. This indicator is often cited as evidence that workers of the future are likely to be overwhelmed unless current commitments are reduced (see Concord Coalition, 1993).

In one sense, the old-age dependency ratio may understate the implications of population aging. It does not capture the relative growth of the very old population, the elderly group with the highest health care and social support costs. Moreover, if middle series Census Bureau and intermediate Social Security mortality assumptions are substantially lower than actual experience, then the overall costs of elder support may be considerably larger.

On the other hand, analysis based on the "overall dependency ratio" (also called the "total support ratio"), which includes children under 18 and elderly persons as "dependent" populations, leads to different conclusions (Crown, 1985). Because the proportion of the population under 18 is expected to decline, during the next 65 years the overall dependency ratio is not projected to exceed the levels it attained in 1965 (83:100). (From 2030 through 2050, the total dependency ratio is projected to be below 78:100.) While acknowledging that the composition of governmental and private spending for children and elderly persons is different, plainly analysis that includes this broader dependency ratio does not lead to the automatic conclusion that changing demographics will overwhelm the nation's ability to respond to the retirement needs of future generations (Crown, 1985; Kingson & Berkowitz, 1993). Neither does it suggest that the nation will necessarily be able to meet these needs, since so much depends on factors such as future productivity and the composition of the work force (National Academy on Aging, 1994).

Diversity of the Baby-Boom Cohorts

Planning for the retirement and long-term care of baby boomers should proceed with an understanding of their diversity (Kingson, 1992; Light, 1988; National Academy on Aging, 1994). Considering baby boomers as a homogeneous group would provide an inaccurate basis for public policy, potentially of great risk to the more economically and socially vulnerable members of the baby-boom cohorts in their old age. Baby boomers differ by 19 years of birth, with the younger members of the boom more likely to feel the pinch of benefit reductions (Bouvier & DeVita, 1991; Congressional Budget Office, 1993; Light, 1988). Conversely, they are likely to reap greater returns from long-term economic growth. They differ, of course, by race and ethnicity, with roughly 18 million baby boomers–including approximately 9.5 million African-Americans, 6.1 million Hispanics, and 2.8 million people of other races[2]–currently classified as "minorities at risk," meaning, among other things, that they are more likely to enter old age with limited financial resources (Kingson, 1992). Within racial and ethnic groups there are also differences; for example, among Hispanics,

Puerto Ricans tend to be the least well-off, Chicanos are in the middle, and Cubans are the most well-off (Torres-Gil, 1986). They differ by education; even though baby boomers have benefited from more education than previous generations (with nearly one quarter graduating from college), more than 3 *million* have not gone beyond the eighth grade (Siegel, 1989).

And, of course, they differ by employment and income. A recent Congressional Budget Office report indicates that they have earnings that at least parallel those of their parents' cohorts at similar points in their lives. However, the progress of the baby boomers falls short of their expectations (Levy, 1987), because their working years have coincided with the slowed economic growth of the last several decades. Since the mid 1970s, the American income distribution has become more unequal, a trend that is reflected among baby boomers, with one in five having family incomes below $14,626 in 1990 and one in five having family incomes above $55,768 (Lewin-VHI, Inc., 1994).

Having experienced more favorable labor market circumstances than younger baby boomers, those born from 1946 to 1954 will likely accrue higher rates of retirement savings in the form of a pension from their employer, Social Security, housing wealth, and other assets. They are likely to be in a better position to fund portions of their long-term care from housing equity (see Apgar et al., 1990).

The racial and economic diversity of these cohorts points to a growing need to plan service systems that are sensitive to this diversity. It is particularly important to recognize that many among minorities at risk "will be at particular risk for social dislocation and stress" during their old age, and they will experience "higher rates of age-specific diseases and disability that reflect substandard medical care and the hardships and dangers of high-risk employment and social environments earlier in the life course" (National Academy on Aging, 1994, p. 21).

Changes in the family. Diversity and change are particularly central to the family life of baby boomers. As a group, their family life is characterized by changes in the institution of marriage and the family, including a diversity in the forms of "family," increased divorce and single-parenthood, fewer children, changes in patterns of caregiving to children, increasingly complex relationships with kin networks, and the growth of three- and four-generation families. A higher proportion (10%) relative to their parents' generation (5%) will never marry (U.S. House of Representatives, 1987). About half of the marriages of baby boomers are expected to end in divorce; but three quarters are expected to remarry (Cherlin & Furstenberg, 1982). Thus, kinship patterns are more complex, and with this complexity comes questions of who is responsible for parental and step-parental care (Hagestad, 1986) and some evidence of a weakening in filial obligation in blended families (National Academy on Aging, 1994).

Fewer children, the increased labor-force participation of women, and the greater likelihood of their parents living longer may constrain the availability of informal support for many aged baby boomers. This may be partially offset by the presence of more siblings. Again, some may do fine. Others, such as divorced single men, who are more likely to become isolated from their children, may be at substantial risk. Low-income single parents among the baby-boom cohorts will likely be at great risk. Their children are substantially more likely to receive less than adequate health care, education, and preparation for productive employment–which has implications for their future productivity as a group and which, on an individual level, may affect their ability to provide care or financial support to their parents as they age.

The old age of baby boomers may coincide with a lessening of family-provided long-term care. This raises important issues since the family is currently the source of roughly 80% of the long-term care to the disabled old (National Academy on Aging, 1994). There is a need for increased understanding of how public interventions and employment policies interact to both support and/or reduce family support, and policy development must take seriously the possibility that changes that have taken place in the family may restrict the capacity of families to provide care.

Retirement resources. The ability of baby boomers to finance their long-term care needs either through public and private pensions, savings, or purchase of long-term care insurance policies will depend heavily on the adequacy of available retirement resources. Some analysts suggest that, on average, baby boomers will enjoy a standard of living in retirement that is at least equal to and probably better than that of today's elders (Congressional Budget Office, 1993; Lewin-VHI, Inc., 1994). But others point out that, while this may be so, they may also experience very substantial declines in their preretirement standards of living (Bemheim, 1994). Moreover, personal savings generally fall short of what is needed to maintain pre-retirement living standards upon retirement.

Social Security is likely to remain the central source of income for older people in the United States. A recent simulation (Lewin-VHI, Inc., 1994) suggests that, in the aggregate, Social Security will account for about 38% of retirement income in 2030, with pension income accounting for 24%, asset income 23%, and earnings 14%. Social Security will be a more important source of income for low- and moderate-income retirees, with 56% of beneficiaries relying on it for at least half their income in 2030. Income from "private pensions is likely to remain [important], particularly for upper income baby boomers, and will gain in importance for women" (Congressional Budget Office, 1993, p. 39). Older baby boomers, so far, have done better than the younger ones to the extent that they have somewhat higher rates of participation in employer pensions (see Woods, 1989).

The risk of poverty and near poverty in their old age will be greatest for those currently at economic risk, especially single parents, the marginally employed, and nonhomeowners. There is also agreement that those who are or become single and those who sustain large health care costs as well as minorities, very old women, and single persons are at substantially greater risk in old age (Lewin-VHI, Inc., 1994; Kingson, 1992; Congressional Budget Office, 1993; National Academy on Aging, 1994). The Lewin-VHI simulations point to an emerging underclass of baby boomers–about four million in 2030–with incomes below 150% of poverty, 85% of whom will be separated, divorced, or never married.

As the retirement income prospects of baby boomers are affected by uncertainties associated with changes in benefit policy, the economy, employment prospects in old age, and savings behavior, it is reasonable to expect much diversity in their standards of living and in their ability to finance their health and long-term care needs. Those facing a retirement of economic deprivation will be dependent on family and public programs to meet their long-term care needs. Without changes in our national policy, long-term care will also likely pose great risk for the more financially secure.

The Growing Risk of Long-Term Care

Given "current age patterns of activity limitation, an average of 12.8 years out of current life expectancy at birth of 75.0 would be spent with some degree of activity limitation" and "an average of 6.9 of the 16.9 years remaining at age 65" (Institute of Medicine, 1991, p. 61).

Diverse long-term care needs. Today's elderly population presents a heterogeneous picture with respect to its health status and care needs and the same can be expected of baby boomers. Cross-sectional data from the 1985 National Health Interview Survey indicate that 5.1 percent of persons under 18, 8.4 percent of persons 18-44, 23.4 percent of persons 45-64, and 39.6 percent of persons 65 and over experience some activity limitations (Institute of Medicine, 1991). While only five percent of the elderly live in nursing homes on any given day, "persons aged 65 years have about a 40 percent chance of spending some time in a nursing home before they die"–the probability is "higher for women . . . than for men" (Kane & Kane, 1990, p. 423). Old age does not, however, signal the beginning of a uniformly downward trend, from good to bad health, and this is likely to remain the case in the future. Older people go through a variety of health transitions. Setbacks to independent living such as broken hips may be followed by improved functioning. Moreover, functional incapacities can be forestalled, prevented, improved and even reversed by lifestyle interventions, rehabilitation, social services, and proper medical care. Research and new technology hold the promise of further progress along this line.

Growing cost of long-term care. Simulations using the Brookings-ICF Long-Term Care Model provide a basis for estimating the numbers of baby boomers in need of community- and institutionally based long-term care and related costs. Base case simulations project 3.6 million elderly nursing home residents and another 7.4 million elderly persons using home care in 2018, the great bulk of whom will not be baby boomers (Weiner, Illston, & Hanley, 1994). Simple extrapolation using the Brookings data and 1992 Census projections suggests that 5.5 million people will be in nursing homes and 11.4 million will be using home care in 2040, the large majority of whom will be baby boomers (see Table 1).[3]

Base case simulations suggest that long-term care costs will grow from $75 billion per year in 1993 to $168 billion in 2018. Extrapolating to 2048, $509 billion will be spent on long-term care (Weiner, Illston, & Hanley, 1994). "Assuming the economy grows at a real rate of 2.5% a year, long-term care will less than double as a percentage of GDP," from 1.21% in 1993 to 2.14% in 2048 (Weiner, Illston, & Hanley, 1994, p. 41). Assuming 1.5% real growth per year, the elderly's long-term care expenditures will nearly triple by 2048 as a percentage of GDP, whereas if the economy averages real growth of 3.5% per year (high growth assumption), expenditures will be only marginally higher in 2048 (Weiner, Illston, & Hanley, 1994).

Baby-boom cohorts may experience lower rates of age-specific chronic illness because higher levels of educational attainment are often associated with more "healthful" behavior (U.S. House of Representatives, 1987) and because, on average, they have been less exposed to the risks associated with physical labor. Basic research may reduce various risks and, along with technological innovation, make chronic illness more manageable. But even so, under all plausible scenarios, more people than today will need long-term care and public and private long-term care costs will increase substantially.

Slowed Growth and Economic Uncertainty

Awareness of economic uncertainty and change influences and constrains long-term care policy discussions. National savings during

Table 1. Estimates of Long-Term Care Costs and Usage to 2050

	1993	2018	2040	2048	2050
65+ Population	32.8 million[a]	49.2 million[b]	75.6 million[a]		78.9 million[a]
85+ Population	3.4 million[a]	6.2 million[b]	13.2 million[a]		17.7 million[a]
Nursing Home Population Brookings-ICF Model[b]	2.2 million	3.6 million			
Rough Extrapolation of Nursing Home Population[c]			5.5 million[c]		5.8 million[d]
Home Care Usage—Brookings-ICF Model[b]	5.2 million	7.4 million			
Rough Extrapolation of Home Care Usage			11.4 million[c]		11.7 million[d]
Total Long-Term Care Expenditures (1993 dollars)[b]	$75 billion	$168 billion		$509 billion	
Total Long-Term Care Expenditures as a percent of gross domestic product[b]	1.21%	1.55%		2.14%	
Public Long-Term Care Expenditures as a percent of gross domestic product[b]	0.65%	0.77%		1.07%	

[a] Day, J.C. (1992), *Current Population Reports*, Table 2.

[b] Wiener, J.M. et al. (1994), *Sharing the Burden*, pp. 34-41, Tables 2-4, Figures 2-2, 2-3.

[c] Estimates assume that the nursing home population and the home care usage population (as projected in the Brookings-ICF model for 2018) will grow by the rate of increase in the projected 65 and over population from 2020 to 2040. Estimates do not adjust for projected changes in the age composition of the elderly population and assume no changes in disability rates for the elderly after 2018.

[d] Estimates assume the same as in footnote "c" except that they are inclusive of the period from 2020 to 2050 instead of 2020 to 2040.

1983-92 dropped as a percentage of net national product to an average of 3.3%. The percent of children under 18 years old who lived in households below the official U.S. poverty threshold rose from 14.4% in 1973 to 22% in 1993. Slowed wage growth threatens the country's ability to pay for the growing costs of aging baby boomers. Health care expenditures have been increasing at a rapid rate, from 7.4% of the nation's gross national product in 1970 to 13.2% in 1991. Medicare's Hospital Insurance program is projected to run out of funds in 2002, and costs are rapidly growing in Medicare's Supplementary Medical Insurance program and in Medicaid. And there is growing recognition of the need to shore up Social Security's long-term financing.

WAYS OF THINKING ABOUT LONG-TERM CARE TRANSFERS

While public services and public expenditures are a critical part of the long-term care system, private exchanges of care are the foundation of the nation's long-term care system. Recognizing the role of informal care focuses more attention on long-term care as a multidimensional risk, of particular concern to women.

Public and Private Financial Exchanges

Public and private cash payments for nursing home and home health care are arguably the most visible long-term care transfers, representing a $70 billion expenditure in 1991. About six times as much is spent on nursing home care as on home care, $60 billion compared to $10 billion in 1991. The Medicaid program pays for roughly one half of all nursing home care and a quarter of home care expenses. The bulk of long-term care services are funded by private sources, primarily by out-of-pocket payments, which accounted for nearly 40% of all long-term care payments in 1991.

These highly visible long-term care transfers dominate long-term care policy discussions. Alarm is often expressed about the growing cost of Medicaid and at seemingly perverse incentives that may encourage middle-class households to transfer or spend down assets to obtain Medicaid eligibility. Federal budget analysts target the rising cost of Medicare's home health and institutionally based rehabilitation benefits. The nursing home industry and home care providers, in turn, carefully monitor the potential effects of new legislation and budgetary and regulatory change. Advocates stress the need for access to a continuum of care and note the financial devastation that chronic illness and related out-of-pocket expenses can visit on the old.

Private Exchanges of Time

Although less recognized as an explicit transfer, the work of families and friends is often the source of critical nonmonetized, long-term care services. This includes time spent negotiating the complex array of health and long-term care services, house-cleaning, preparing meals, shopping, and assisting with personal care.

Caregiving has many of the same attributes as public income and health care transfers, including tangible worth. Assigning a value of $6 an hour to housework, childcare and other caregiving activities, James Morgan (1983) estimated that families transferred the equivalent of 30% of the gross national product in 1979. Absent these informal caregivers, functionally disabled elders must either do without certain services or pay for them with public or personal funds.

The distribution of the benefits and costs of caregiving vary, depending upon whether they are examined at one point in time or over time. From a cross-sectional perspective, long-term caregiving can be viewed primarily as a transfer from able and often younger family members, to older and more disabled members. In other words, older people generally receive the benefit of care and younger spouses, siblings, children, or friends pay the cost in time taken from paid work, leisure, or other caregiving. But from a longitudinal perspective, caregiving is part of the reciprocity of giving and receiving that varies over the lives of individuals and cohorts, and creates the ties that bind family and community life (see Kingson, Hirshorn, & Cornman, 1986). When viewed from this longitudinal perspective, receipt of care represents a return for care that was previously given by the recipient, and is part of a lifelong exchange.

Giving and Receiving Long-Term Care as a Women's Issue

Thinking about long-term care as a women's issue helps clarify why the invisibility of much caregiving work within the context of the family and the parallel devaluation of formal caregiving need to emerge as explicit public policy issues. Informal caregiving is generally an afterthought of public policy discussions on long-term care. Policy planners express concern about caregiver stress and researchers note costs, in the form of lost wages and smaller retirement benefits, for those caregivers who must compromise their employment efforts. But serious public policy attention is rarely given to such concerns. Why? The answer can be found in assumptions about who is expected to give care and in the value assigned to this care. Laura Olson notes, "[N]ot only have more females added care of the superannuated to their productive and reproductive roles, but, in addition, these efforts tend to be both invisible and undervalued" (1994, p. 13).

According to Elaine Brody (1990), "Women represent over 70% of all caregivers, including adult daughters (30%), wives (23%), and other female relatives, many of whom are daughter-in-laws and sisters (20%)." Frail elderly men generally rely on spouses, and frail elderly women, on adult children, especially daughters where present (Olson, 1994). Plainly, the risk of being a lifelong caregiver (see Rimmer, 1983)–first to children, to young or middle-aged disabled family members, to aged parents or in-laws, and to an aged spouse–is much greater for women than men. Thus, the costs associated with caregiving–stress, lost career mobility, smaller wages, lost leisure, reductions in retirement benefits–accrue disproportionately to women.

Women also bear the greatest risk of being paid low wages as part of the formal caregiving system. A high proportion of home care and nursing home employees are middle aged, minority women, often with limited education. Almost 90% of nurses' aides and other paraprofessionals in nursing homes are women, and in 1986 the average salary for nurses' aides was under $4 per hour (Olson, 1994). Low wages compromise the well-being of these caregivers and can affect quality of care to elders, usually women.

And finally, older women are at greater risk than men. Compared to men, older women also have higher rates of functional limitations at ages 65-74, 75-84, and over 85, are more likely to be single, have fewer available informal caregivers, live longer, and have lower incomes. Consequently, their risk of institutionalization is greater and, once institutionalized, they are likely to be in institutions for a longer period than men (Conner, 1992).

COMPETING PERSPECTIVES

The Generational Equity/Crisis Perspective

The generational equity/crisis perspective raises important questions about fairness in the distribution of public resources between younger and older age groups and cohorts. It highlights concerns about the ability of tomorrow's younger and middle-aged workers to meet existing federal promises to aging baby-boom cohorts. Given large federal deficits, declining national savings, and what are viewed as unrealistically large governmental commitments to older populations, there is little justification for new spending for universal long-term care. In fact, existing public entitlements serving today's elderly are viewed as unsustainable in the future, a cause of budget deficits, poorly targeted to persons in need, and undermining the economy and the well-being of future generations–thus the "crisis." The baby boomers from this point of view are headed for a disastrous retirement because they are not saving enough for their retirement years, and not investing enough to secure a strong economy for their children.

Some espousing variants of this view propose substantially reducing the size of entitlements (and with it the public sector), targeting public resources more toward low-income elderly persons, and encouraging more private savings and investment (Concord Coalition, 1993). Others are concerned that entitlements directed at the old are restricting the ability of the Congress to address other important concerns. In this regard, some consider that redirecting entitlements away from today's and tomorrow's elderly would be a means of providing more for children. These issues and others related to preparing for the future, form the agenda of a movement that calls for "generational equity."

Adherents of this view can be found across the entire spectrum of political opinion in the United States. Even so, as articulated by its most vocal adherents (e.g., Concord Coalition, 1993; Kotlikoff, 1992; Longman, 1987; Petersen & Howe, 1989), the generational equity/crisis perspective represents, most fundamentally, a recasting of the traditional conservative political stance with respect to the proper role of government in a market economy (Marmor, Mashaw, & Harvey, 1990). Thus, the subtext of the generational equity debate is centered on differences regarding the proper role of government and the public versus the private provision of resources, not fairness between generations (see Minkler, 1986).

The Generational Investment/Gradual Adjustment Perspective

The generational investment/gradual adjustment perspective defines the aging of the baby-boom cohorts as a surmountable challenge, requiring adjustments–quite possibly reductions–in existing retirement and health policies and programs. In contrast to the generational equity view, the generational investment/gradual adjustment view is that the claim that older cohorts have to a reasonable return (in the form of retirement and health benefits) arises from their prior investments in the economy and in the well-being of younger cohorts (see National Academy on Aging, 1994). It defines public benefits as an outgrowth of the interdependence and reciprocity of generations, part of a complex set of exchanges–some public and some private–that occur over the lives of individuals and cohorts. It implies that benefits from policies directed at the old flow across cohorts; that is, are not restricted only to the old (see Kingson, Hirshorn, & Cornman, 1986). While recognizing that such claims must be balanced against other social and economic needs and may require reductions in benefits to older people, this perspective reinforces public interventions such as Social Security and Medicare, and is open to considering new public long-term care initiatives.

This perspective also builds its analysis on a recognition of the heterogeneity of older populations, a theme that is consistent with differentiating among elderly populations with respect to the distribution of social benefits and obligations. From this perspective, increased investment in the economy is needed now to avoid problems in the future and, as in the past, adjustments will need to be made in Social Security, Medicare, and related problems in response to changing economics and demographics.

This view can be seen as serving the function–good or bad depending on one's perspective–of supporting existing programs and policies and reducing the likelihood that serious attention will be given to radical proposals such as means testing or privatizing Social Security. Thus, to its critics, generational investment is less a goal than a rationale for maintaining the elder service structure.

Relevant Facts, Problems and Solutions: Conflicting Views

There is little disagreement over the basic trends associated with the aging of the baby-boom cohorts. All agree that the numbers of old and the very old will grow rapidly; that persons under 18 are becoming a smaller portion of the population; that the aging of baby boomers will strain the public and private retirement and health care systems; and that there will be a substantial demand for long-term care.

Differences arise over the emphasis placed on various facts and the inferences drawn. Consistent with the generational investment/gradual adjustment perspective is the idea that population aging represents a challenge, one that exists because of successful investments throughout the century in the public's health and standard of living (Kingson, Hirshorn, & Cornman, 1986). The challenge represented by the aging of the baby-boom generation does not necessarily require radical adjustments in social policy as much as prudent planning and careful investment of public and private resources. Thus, increased investment in research designed to reduce frailty and delay the onset of chronic illnesses is urged by some (Butler & Perry, 1989, p. 84). Similarly, investment in the productive capacity of the young can be viewed as a fundamental form of societal savings, and "one which properly generates returns for young and old alike" (National Academy on Aging, 1994).

In contrast, the generational equity/crisis perspective views these population trends with alarm. They may represent a success, but they are clearly a huge worry. Recognition of changing demographics is generally the starting point for warnings of dire circumstances that will follow if radical change does not take place quickly (see Longman, 1987; Petersen & Howe, 1989). Phillip Longman warns that the "likely result of these trends and the retirement expectations of the baby boomers," unless many fundamental trends are soon reversed, will be a war between young and old (Longman, 1987, p. 2). Peter G. Petersen and Neil Howe (1989) express concerns about declining savings and investment and the imprudent use of resources. Without change, they argue, a crisis cannot be averted merely by future economic growth.

This perspective often draws on the changing dependency ratio, suggesting that commitments to future cohorts of the old will be unsustainable as the ratio changes. Moreover, given the possibilities of there being larger older populations than currently estimated, the situation might be worse.

The generational investment/gradual adjustment view is cautiously optimistic that, with significant adjustments, the challenge posed by the aging of the baby-boom cohorts can be overcome. In contrast, the generational equity/crisis view is deeply pessimistic about future possibilities without more fundamental change. Both views consider economic growth as critical to the well-being of all age groups as the population ages. But where the generational investment view simply calls for investment and implicitly suggests that the country can "muddle through"; the generational equity view argues that adequate investment is not possible without reducing public commitments directed at future cohorts of the old.

The generational equity perspective builds, in part, on a growing awareness of the diverse economic circumstances of the old, especially today's old. The needs of low-income elders are often acknowledged as an appropriate target of government intervention, but often primarily as a byproduct of a position advocating shifting from a universal to a means-tested selective base for benefits. Also, the generational equity framework often gives rise to stereotypes of the old (presumably tomorrow's old, too) as "greedy geezers" or, incorrectly, as the most well-off among Americans. The presumption here is that a large proportion of elders are receiving (or will receive) public benefits that they neither need or deserve. From within this perspective, Social Security and other entitlements for the elderly are distributively perverse, meaning that they subsidize higher-income persons while neglecting the needs of lower-income persons. Also, from this perspective, it is unfair to baby boomers that programs such as Social Security transfer resources from today's young to today's old, and will not provide baby boomers with a fair rate of return. And federal deficits throw generational accounts further out of balance (Kotlikoff, 1992).

Academic gerontologists have been in the forefront of identifying the changing status and diversity of elderly populations. James Schulz (1976) noted that aged populations are not an economically homogeneous group, and Robert Hudson and Robert Binstock (1976) made similar observations concerning voting and other political behavior. Generational investment/gradual adjustment analyses generally recognize these truths and the need to plan for many different groups of baby boomers, especially those at greatest risk (see Bouvier & De Vita, 1991; Kingson, 1992; Lewin-VHI, 1994; Light, 1988; National Academy on Aging, 1994). But, unlike the generational equity framework, the generational investment view does not consider them to be a reason to abandon commitments to social insurance, though such knowledge may lead to increased targeting (e.g., taxation of Social Security) within a social insurance framework.

These perspectives emphasize different distributive consequences of long-term care for the baby-boom cohorts. The generational equity/crisis perspective places more emphasis on the growing burden to younger taxpayers and the potential of further public commitments to undermine economic growth. Long-term care services are clearly defined as a transfer from young to old. Family care is assumed, with little attention paid to the implications of gender-specific costs and benefits among family members. In contrast, the generational investment perspective approaches long-term care policy in a way that places more emphasis on the distributive costs of not providing care and less emphasis on the costs to taxpayers of how to pay for such care. Whereas the generational equity/crisis perspective is challenged to justify placing an increased burden on families and ignoring important women's issues, the generational investment perspective is challenged to justify the distributive consequences of taxes that will need to be raised for new long-term care interventions. The generational equity perspective needs to acknowledge that one way or another we will need to pay for the long-term care of the baby boomers–either through increased taxes, by placing a greater financial burden on individuals, or by imposing more stress on family systems: In other words, there is no free lunch. Similarly, the generational equity perspective needs to acknowledge that public interventions may be costly, and it needs to justify new expenditures in a period of large projected deficits: In other words, there is no free lunch. No matter how the long-term care policy issue for the baby-boom cohorts is framed, there is no escaping the need to approach this issue with a recognition that there are real costs–public, private, familial, and gender-related–for anything that we choose to do or not do.

To summarize, these two perspectives proceed from different assumptions about the role of social programs in protecting the well-being of the population, and these differences influence the facts that are marshaled and the framing of the problems of long-term care for the baby-boom cohorts. The generational equity perspective is consonant with a smaller public sector and generally assumes that individuals should be personally responsible for the various risks associated with old age. From this point of view, the purposes of government programs should be to reduce existing poverty or provide critical services such as long-term care only when there is clear financial need. As regards specific long-term care interventions for the baby-boom cohorts, they are most consistent with proposals to expand private savings for long-term care contingencies and private long-term insurance and, secondarily, with proposals to expand means-tested provisions. But from the generational investment perspective, social interventions should assist citizens to plan for risks, and should prevent poverty. This perspective is plainly more consistent with proposals to create new universal services through a traditional social insurance approach or through a universal block grant, such as those discussed in the Clinton health care reform effort.

ENDNOTES

1. In the context of the United States, the term "white non-Hispanic population" refers to persons who are considered among the "majority" population.
2. These figures are not additive because Hispanics are distributed across all racial categories.
3. This is a very crude estimate since it does not take potential changes in disability and rates and policy into account nor does it adjust for age-specific risks of needing long-term care.

REFERENCES

Apgar, Jr., W. C., DiPasquale, D., McArdle, N., & Olson, N. (1990). *The state of the nation's housing 1989*. Cambridge, MA: Joint Center for Housing Studies, Harvard University.

Board of Trustees, Federal Old-Age and Survivors Insurance and Disability Insurance Trust Funds (1994). *1994 Annual Report of the Federal Old-Age and Survivors Insurance and Disability Insurance Trust Funds*. Washington, DC: U.S. Government Printing Office.

Bouvier, L. F., & De Vita, C. J. (1991). *The baby boom–Entering midlife*. Washington, DC: Population Reference Bureau.
Brody, E. (1990). *Women in the middle: Their parent-care years*. New York, NY: Springer Publishing Company.
Butler, R. N., & Perry, D. (1989). Aging research needed before baby boomers become the largest 'Medicare generation' in American history. *The Generational Journal, 2* (1), 84-85.
Cherlin, A., & Furstenberg, Jr., F. (1982). *The shape of the American family in the year 2000: Trends Analysis Program*. Washington, DC: American Council of Life Insurance.
Concord Coalition (1993). *The zero deficit plan*. Washington, DC: Author.
Congressional Budget Office (1993, September). *Baby boomers in retirement: An early perspective*. Washington, DC: Author.
Conner, K. A. (1992). *Aging America: Issues facing an aging society*. Englewood Cliffs, NJ: Prentice Hall.
Crown, W. H. (April, 1985). Some thoughts on reformulating the dependency ratio. *The Gerontologist, 24*, 166-171.
Day, J. C. (1992). Population projections of the United States, by age, sex, race, and Hispanic origin: 1992 to 2050. *Current Population Reports*, Series P25, No. 1092. Washington, DC: U.S. Government Printing Office.
Douglas, B. (1994, May 4). *The adequacy of savings for retirement: Are the baby boomers on track*? Paper prepared for policy forum sponsored by the Employee Benefit Research Institute, Washington, DC.
Hagestad, G. O. (1986). The family: Women and grandparents as kin-keepers. In Pifer, A., & Bronte, L. (Eds.) *Our aging society: paradox and promise* (pp. 141-160). New York: W.W. Norton & Company.
Hudson, R. B., & Binstock, R. H. (1976). Political systems and aging. In Binstock, R. H., & Shanas, E. (Eds.), *Handbook of aging and the social sciences* (pp. 511-535). New York: Van Nostrand Reinhold Company.
Institute of Medicine (1993). *Disability in America: Toward a national agenda for prevention*. Washington, DC: National Academy of Sciences.
Kane, R. L., & Kane, R. A. (1990). Health care for older people: Organizational and policy issues. In Binstock, R. H., & George, L. K. (Eds.), *Handbook of aging and the social sciences* (pp. 415-445). San Diego: Academic Press.
Kingson, E. R. (1992, April). *The diversity of the baby boom generation: Implications for their retirement years*. Washington, DC: American Association of Retired Persons, Forecasting and Environmental Scanning Division.
Kingson, E. R., & Berkowitz, E. D. (1993). *Social Security and Medicare: A policy primer*. Westport, CT: Auburn House.
Kingson, E. R., Hirshorn, B. A., & Cornman, J. M. (1986). *Ties that bind: The interdependence of generations*. Cabin John, MD: Seven Locks Press.
Kotlikoff, L. J. (1992). *Generational accounting: Knowing who pays, and when, for what we spend*. New York: The Free Press.
Levy, F. (1987). *Dollars and dreams: The changing American income distribution*. New York: Russell Sage Foundation.

Lewin-VHI Inc. (1994). *Aging baby boomers: How secure is their economic future?* Washington, DC: American Association of Retired Persons, Forecasting and Environmental Scanning Division.

Light, P. C. (1988). *Baby boomers.* New York: W.W. Norton & Company.

Longman, P. (1987). *Born to pay: The new politics of aging in America.* Boston: Houghton Mifflin Company.

Manton, K. G., Corder, L. S., & Stallard, E. (1993, July). Estimates of change in chronic disability and institutional incidence and prevalence rates in the U.S. elderly population from the 1982, 1984, and 1989 National Long Term Care Survey. *Journal of Gerontology: Social Sciences, 48*, 4 (July 1993), S153-S166.

Marmor, T. R., Mashaw, J. L., & Harvey, P. L. (1990). *Misunderstood welfare state: Persistent myths, enduring realities.* New York: Basic Books.

Minkler, M. (1986). "Generational equity" and the new victim blaming: An emerging public policy issue. *International Journal of Health Services, 16,* 539-551.

Morgan, J. N. (1983). The redistribution of income by families and institutions and emergency help patterns. In Duncan, G. J., & Morgan, H. M. (Eds.), *Five thousand American families: Patterns of economic progress, vol. 10, Analysis of the first thirteen years of the panel of income dynamics* (pp. 26-42). Ann Arbor, MI: Institute for Social Research, University of Michigan.

National Academy on Aging (1994, July). *Old age in the 21st century.* Washington, DC: National Academy on Aging.

Olson, L. K. (1994). *The graying of the world: Who will care for the frail elderly?* New York: The Haworth Press, Inc.

Petersen, P. G., & Howe, N. (1989). *On borrowed time.* San Francisco: Institute for Contemporary Studies.

Rimmer, L. (1983). The economics of work and caring. In Finch, J., & Groves, D. (eds.), *A labor of love: Women, work and caring* (pp. 131-147). London: Routledge and Keagan Paul.

Schulz, J. H. (1976). *The economics of aging.* Belmont, CA: Wadsworth Publishing Company.

Siegel, P. M. (1989). Educational attainment in the United States: March 1982 to 1985. *Current Population Reports*, U.S. Bureau of the Census, Series P-20, No. 415. Washington, DC: U.S. Government Printing Office.

Soldo, B. J., & Agree, A. M. (1988, September). America's elderly. In *Population Bulletin*, Vol. 43, No. 3. Washington, DC: Population Reference Bureau.

Torres-Gil, F. (1986). Hispanics: A special challenge. In Pifer, A. & Bronte, L. (Eds.), *Our aging society: Paradox and promise* (pp. 219-242). W.W. Norton & Company.

U.S. House of Representatives, Committee on Ways and Means. (1987, August 25). *Retirement income for an aging society.* Washington, DC: U.S. Government Printing Office.

Verbrugge, L. M. (1991). *Proceedings of the second conference of the National Academy of Social Insurance.* Washington, DC: National Academy of Social Insurance.

Wiener, J. M., Illston, L. H., & Hanley, R. J. (1994). *Sharing the burden: Strategies for public and private long-term care insurance*. Washington, DC: The Brookings Institution.

Woods, J. R. (1989, October). Pension coverage among private wage and salary workers: Preliminary findings from the 1988 survey of employee benefits. *Social Security Bulletin*.

Changes in Health, Mortality, and Disability and Their Impact on Long-Term Care Needs

Kenneth G. Manton, PhD
Eric Stallard, ASA, MAAA

Duke University
Durham, North Carolina

SUMMARY. The need for long-term care is driven both by the growth of the elderly population and changes in the age relations of morbidity, disability, and mortality. Data show these relations changed in the U.S. elderly population from 1982 to 1989. Chronic disability prevalence declined between the 1982 and 1989 U.S. National Long Term Care Surveys. Among those impaired, many persons using personal assistance to meet their needs shifted to the use of assisted housing and special equipment. The relation of these

---

Kenneth G. Manton is Research Professor at the Center for Demographic Studies and Research Director of Demographic Studies, Duke University, as well as Medical Research Professor at Duke University Medical Center's Department of Community and Family Medicine. Dr. Manton is also a Senior Fellow of the Duke University Medical Center's Center for the Study of Aging and Human Development. Eric Stallard is Research Professor at the Center for Demographic Studies; he is an Associate of the Society of Actuaries and a Member of the American Academy of Actuaries.

The research on which this article is based was supported by Grant Nos. AG07025, AG07469, and AG07198 from the National Institute on Aging.

The authors can be contacted care of the Center for Demographic Studies, Duke University, 2117 Campus Drive, Durham, NC 27708.

[Haworth co-indexing entry note]: "Changes in Health, Mortality, and Disability and Their Impact on Long-Term Care Needs." Manton, Kenneth G. and Eric Stallard. Co-published simultaneously in *Journal of Aging & Social Policy* (The Haworth Press, Inc.) Vol. 7, No. 3/4, 1996, pp. 25-52; and: *From Nursing Homes to Home Care* (ed: Marie E. Cowart and Jill Quadagno) The Haworth Press, Inc., 1996, pp. 25-52. Single or multiple copies of this article are available from The Haworth Document Delivery Service [1-800-342-9678, 9:00 a.m. - 5:00 p.m. (EST)].

trends to other changes–such as the increasing educational level of the elderly population–is examined to estimate how future changes in disability and morbidity may affect the demand for long-term care. Disabilities at specific times as well as their transition rates were examined to determine how long individuals need long-term care. The analyses suggest that, while the amount of long-term care services needed will increase rapidly, the types and amounts of services used by the U.S. elderly population will undergo significant change. *[Article copies available from The Haworth Document Delivery Service: 1-800-342-9678.]*

Proposals have been made to provide long-term care to the U.S. chronically disabled population. In this article, the focus is on the elderly chronically disabled. Despite the growth of the U.S. elderly population, no federal long-term care policy has been implemented because of its cost. Implementation of Medicare long-term care benefits could cost from $38 billion (the Pepper Commission) to $43 billion (the Steelman Commission). An actuarial evaluation suggests costs could be $35.8 billion in fiscal year 1996, increasing to $53.9 billion in fiscal year 2000. This article does not propose a policy but examines the health and social conditions of the U.S. elderly population to see if assumptions made in long-term care proposals are valid. If conditions change, this may open new policy options.

There are changes in the health of the elderly (Manton, Corder, & Stallard 1993a, 1993b; Manton, Stallard, & Corder, 1995), their social and economic status, biomedical knowledge of how health changes at late ages, and in the private and public housing and health care markets. The data suggest that declines in chronic morbidity and disability are long-standing. Stroke mortality has decreased since 1925 (Lanska & Mi, 1993)–possibly due to regulations regarding livestock feeding that has reduced circulatory disease (Mozar, Bal, & Farag, 1990). Comparing Civil War veterans aged 65 and older in 1910 with World War II veterans also aged 65 and older in 1985, Robert Fogel (1994) found chronic morbidity prevalence declined 6% per decade. Thus, forecasts of the growth of the elderly population and its long-term care needs require reevaluation as well as the optimal mix of strategies to provide these services.

This article examines changes in the health of the U.S. elderly population using the 1982, 1984, and 1989 National Long Term Care Surveys. Both disability prevalence and active life expectancy changes are examined. Second, advances in treatments that improved prognoses and were cost-effective are examined. Third, changes in Medicare use–especially when biomedical advances allow some long-term care needs to be met by interventions in early disease stages–are considered. In these analyses, only the U.S. elderly (65 and older) Medicare population is analyzed.

TRENDS IN HEALTH AND FUNCTIONING AMONG THE ELDERLY

To measure functioning, the prevalence of impairments in activities of daily living, or ADLs (Katz & Akpom, 1976), instrumental activities of daily living, or IADLs (Lawton & Brody, 1969), and institutional residence in the U.S. elderly population were examined. To be chronically disabled, a person had to be unable (or expect to be unable) to perform an ADL without special equipment, or assistance, for 90 or more days. The six ADLs were: bathing, dressing, eating, toileting, getting in/out of bed, and getting around inside. IADL impairment had to result from a physical disability or health problem. IADLs used were: light housework, laundry, meal preparation, grocery shopping, getting around outside, travel, money management, and telephone.

Disability

Table 1 shows the 1989 rates, and the 1982 rates directly standardized to the 1989 age distribution.

The age-adjusted decline in disability is 1.97%, implying 609,000 fewer chronically disabled persons in 1989 than if 1982 rates had not changed–a relative decline of 8.1% (i.e., 22.56%/24.54% = .919). Changes were not uniform. For those with three or more ADLs or in institutions, there are 253,000 fewer disabled persons. Individuals in institutions are screened to be chronically disabled. In 1984, 85.3% of the National Long Term Care Survey institutional population (1,316,021 persons) were in nursing homes (compared to 1,318,300 residents 65 and older in the 1985 National Nursing Home Survey). In 1989, 84.7% of the National Long Term Care Survey institutional population were in nursing homes (1,426,883 persons).

Table 2 shows age and gender specific changes in disability from 1982 to 1989.

The prevalence for males declined 2.84%; for females, 1.28%. Standardized by age and sex, the decline is 1.91%. Male improvements exceed female improvements in all categories except institutions. The largest gender difference is the increase of females with one to two ADLs impaired. The five-to-six ADL impaired and institutionalized groups declined for both genders. The decrease in persons institutionalized, with

TABLE 1: Disability Levels for Persons Aged 65 Years and Older–Percent Distribution and Change, United States 1982 to 1989

Disability Level	(1) Observed 1982	(2) Expected 1989	(3) Observed 1989	(4) Observed Change (3) - (1)	(5) Age Standardized Change (3) - (2)	(6) Age Standardized Change in Population
Nondisabled	76.32	75.46	77.44	1.12	1.97	609,315
IADL	5.33	5.40	4.41	−0.92	−0.99	−306,723
1-2 ADLs	6.46	6.62	6.46	−0.01	−0.16	−49,887
3-4 ADLs	2.72	2.80	3.49	0.78	0.69	213,568
5-6 ADLs	3.48	3.61	2.75	−0.73	−0.90	−265,197
Institutional	5.69	6.11	5.45	−0.23	−0.65	−201,073

NOTES:
Col. (1) - (5): In percent
Col. (2): Age standardized rates; 1982 age specific rates applied to 1989 age specific population distribution.
Col. (6): Age standardized counts; entry in column 5 applied to 1989 population count.

three to four or five to six ADLs impaired, is similar: 0.94% for males and 0.70% for females. Given the greater number of females, their absolute changes are greater.

Two important issues are (1) how rapidly do persons change disability? and (2) do the chronically disabled ever become sufficiently functional again to be "socially autonomous?" Table 3 shows long-term (20-year) changes in disability for persons age 65 who survive to 85.

A significant number of nondisabled persons reach 85 in a nondisabled state (58.3%); also significant numbers of people temporarily lose but then regain functioning. Of survivors to age 85 who had IADL impairments at 65, 45.6% later regained those functions. At most disability levels, significant proportions of survivors to 85 regain function. Those in institutions show little improvement (94.7% die before 85).

Morbidity

Because chronic disability declined from 1982 to 1989, and persons surviving to late ages can preserve or regain function, it is useful to ask what factors underlie those changes and whether their dynamics can be described. Morbidity changes affect chronic disability. Morbidity is often difficult to measure–it may also be difficult to determine the direction of causality. In Table 4 are 1982 and 1989 disease prevalence rates.

Arthritis, circulatory diseases, and dementia rates declined. Prevalence increased for all other types of heart disease, pulmonary problems, and

TABLE 2: Disability Levels for Persons Aged 65 Years and Older, by Sex–Percent Distribution and Change, United States 1982 to 1989

	(1) Observed 1982			(2) Expected 1989			(3) Observed 1989			(4) Change (3)-(2)		
Disability Level	M	F	T	M	F	T	M	F	T	M	F	T
Nondisabled	80.36	73.71	76.32	79.83	72.63	75.53	82.67	73.90	77.44	2.84	1.28	1.91
IADL	4.93	5.58	5.33	5.01	5.64	5.38	3.86	4.77	4.41	−1.15	−0.86	−0.98
1-2 ADLs	5.25	7.25	6.46	5.39	7.40	6.59	4.63	7.69	6.46	−0.76	0.29	−0.13
3-4 ADLs	2.32	2.98	2.72	2.37	3.07	2.79	2.83	3.94	3.50	0.46	0.87	0.70
5-6 ADLS	3.36	3.56	3.48	3.44	3.73	3.61	2.35	3.02	2.75	−1.09	−0.71	−0.86
Institutional	3.78	6.92	5.69	3.97	7.53	6.09	3.66	6.67	5.46	−0.31	−0.86	−0.64

NOTES;
Panels (1) - (4): In percent
Panel (2): Age and sex standardized rates; 1982 age-sex specific rates applied to 1989 age-sex specific population distribution.

fractures. The average number of conditions declined 10.5%–from the 2.56 conditions that would be expected in 1989 if the 1982 age and sex specific rates had not changed–to the average of 2.29 conditions actually observed in 1989. Morbidity declines can also be standardized by disability level, in addition to age and sex. This adjustment produces the same, or larger, changes (compare columns 4 and 6). Column 7 provides t-tests to evaluate differences between columns 3 and 5. Morbidity improved within disability levels. Morbidity has been found to decline within disability level (e.g., those with ADLs only; those with IADLs only; the nondisabled) and in other subgroups (males and females; persons age 85 and over) (Manton, Stallard, & Corder, 1995). There are two reasons why disability standardization did not eliminate morbidity declines. One is that morbidity is associated with disability in general, that is, different diseases may trigger the same disability trajectories. Second, the time between the morbid event and disability may be long, that is, the correlation is strong only if lagged. If medical conditions (e.g., arthritis, dementia, stroke) cause disability, disability prevalence will continue to decline.

Education

One factor affecting morbidity and disability is the educational level of the elderly. The amount of education is related to dementia (e.g., Evans, Scherr, & Cook et al., 1992), mortality, compliance with medical therapy, and the avoidance of risk-factor exposures such as smoking or high fat diets. Furthermore, there may be motivational factors that keep better-educated persons functional, for example, given identical degrees of degenerative joint diseases or osteoarthritis (Hannan, Anderson, Pincus, & Felson, 1992), the better-educated group remains more functional. Osteoarthritis and dementia are two prevalent diseases for which differences in education are important.

Samuel Preston (1992) projected a drop in the proportion of the U.S. population aged 85 to 89 years with low levels of education from 1980 to 2015. For example, 62.1% of males aged 85 to 89 in 1980 had eight or less years of education; by 1995, this drops to 44.4%; by 2015, to 20.0%. For females in the group aged 85 to 89 in 1980, 54.7% had eight years or less of education (in the same group, aged 45 to 49 in the 1940 census, 63.5% had eight years or less of education); by 1995, this drops to 36.5%; by 2015 to 13.7%. Those aged 85 to 89 in 2015 were aged 65 to 69 in 1995. Thus, reductions in 2015 for 85- to 89-year-olds are achieved by 1995 for persons aged 65 to 69, that is, the young-old age group is currently showing rapid changes in education–consistent with the age-specific disability and morbidity declines.

TABLE 3: Twenty-Year Transition Probabilities (in Percent) for Age 65 to 85 Estimated From the 1984 to 1989 NLTCS, With and Without Adjustment, United States

Status at age 65				Status at age 85			
	Nondisabled	IADL Only	1-2 ADLs	3-4 ADLs	5-6 ADLs	Institutional	Dead
Nondisabled	21.8	2.4	4.1	2.5	1.9	4.7	62.6
(excl. dead)	58.3	6.3	11.0	6.6	5.0	12.7	---
IADL Only	8.8	1.2	2.6	1.8	1.3	3.5	80.8
(excl. dead)	45.6	6.5	13.4	9.2	6.9	18.4	---
1-2 ADLs	6.3	1.0	2.3	1.6	1.2	3.4	84.1
(excl. dead)	39.7	6.4	14.2	10.4	7.7	21.7	---
3-4 ADLs	2.5	0.6	1.6	1.3	1.0	2.8	90.1
(excl. dead)	25.3	6.3	16.6	13.4	10.0	28.5	---
5-6 ADLs	2.1	0.4	1.1	0.8	0.6	2.0	93.0
(excl. dead)	29.6	6.0	15.1	11.6	8.9	28.9	---
Institutional	0.6	0.2	0.7	0.4	0.3	3.0	94.7
(excl. dead)	11.4	3.8	12.5	8.1	6.6	57.7	---

Source: Data are from the 1984 and 1989 National Long Term Care Surveys. Estimates are the results of multiplying the five-year transition matrices for ages 65, 70, 75, and 80.

TABLE 4: Total U.S. Noninstitutional Elderly Population; Morbidity Prevalence (in %) From the 1982 and 1989 National Long Term Care Surveys

	(1)	(2)	(3)	(4)	(5)	(6)	(7)
	Observed	Expected	Observed	Change	Expected	Change	t-test
Condition	1982	1989	1989	(3)-(2)	1989	(3)-(5)	(6)
			Percent with Indicated Condition				
1. Arthritis	68.8	70.5	63.1	−7.4	71.1	−8.0	−8.2*
2. Parkinson's	0.8	0.8	1.3	0.5	0.8	0.5	2.6*
3. Diabetes	11.0	11.2	12.4	1.2	11.4	1.0	1.5
4. Cancer	6.2	6.4	5.7	−0.7	6.5	−0.8	−1.6
5. Arteriosclerosis	20.7	21.2	14.9	−6.3	21.4	−6.5	−7.7*
6. Dementia	2.8	2.9	1.7	−1.2	2.9	−1.2	−3.7*
7. Heart Attack	3.7	3.8	3.2	−0.7	3.8	−0.7	−1.8
8. Other Heart	19.5	20.0	22.9	2.9	20.2	2.7	3.2*

9. Hypertension	44.5	45.6	39.5	−6.0	46.0	−6.5	−6.1*
10. Stroke	3.4	3.4	2.6	−0.4	3.4	−0.9	−2.5*
11. Circulation	40.7	41.7	32.1	−9.6	42.1	−10.0	−9.5*
12. Pneumonia	2.9	2.9	4.8	1.8	2.9	1.8	5.3*
13. Bronchitis	9.5	9.8	12.1	2.2	9.8	2.2	3.6*
14. Emphysema	8.6	8.8	6.4	−2.2	8.9	−2.3	−4.3*
15. Asthma	6.5	6.7	6.3	−0.4	6.7	−0.4	−0.8
16. Broken Hip/Fractures	0.5	0.5	0.9	0.4	0.5	0.4	2.9*
			Average number of conditions				
	2.50	2.56	2.29	−0.27	2.58	−0.29	−9.3*
Summary 1 - 16				(−10.5%)		(−11.2%)	

NOTES:

Col. (2): Age and sex standardized rates; 1982 age and sex specific rates applied to 1989 age specific population distribution

Col. (5): Age, sex, and disability standardized rates; 1982 age, sex, and disability specific rates applied to 1989 age, sex, and disability specific population distribution.

Col. (7): *Significant at 0.05 level

Table 5 shows the distributions of disability in 1989 for elderly community residents with less than a high school education and for those with a high school diploma.

The low-education group was 5.73% more likely to be disabled. Most of the excess disability for the low-education group (3.8%) was for those persons with only IADLs (1.9%) or 1 to 2 ADLs (1.9%) impaired. The smallest excess for the low education (0.75%) was for persons with 3 to 4 ADLs impaired. Those with 5 to 6 ADLs impaired contributed 1.2% to the overall excess. The gradient of disability over education is not simple. This may be due to persons with more education, impaired in 3 to 4 ADLs, having greater resources to remain in the community. Overall, in 1989, 44.1% of U.S. community residents aged 65 and older were high school graduates; 55.9% were not. These estimates are lower than in U.S. Bureau of the Census (1992), where 54.9% were high school graduates. These differences may result because education was assessed for a subset of the nondisabled in the NLTCS, who had been disabled at a prior assessment. Because estimates of nondisabled high school graduates in column 3 are low, the differences in columns 4 and 5 are lower bounds to the true effect of education.

In Table 6, high- and low-education groups by age are stratified.

At all ages, the better-educated group had less impairment. Overall differences in the prevalence of chronic disability increases from 2.44% at ages 65 to 74 to 8.97% at 85 and older. Education reduces all levels of disability except for persons with 3 to 4 ADLs at age 65 to 74. A bias in high school graduation rates does *not* occur at age 85 and older. Preston (1992) obtained a graduation rate of 36.3% at ages 85 to 89 in 1990–close

TABLE 5: Disability Levels for Noninstitutional Persons Aged 65 Years and Older, by Education–Percent Distribution, United States 1989

Disability Level	(1) Total	(2) Up to High School	(3) High School Graduate	(4) Difference (3)-(2)	(5) Difference (3)-(1)
Nondisabled	82.01	79.48	85.21	5.73	3.20
IADLs	4.63	5.47	3.57	−1.90	−1.06
1-2 ADLs	6.83	7.68	5.75	−1.93	−1.08
3-4 ADLs	3.70	4.03	3.28	−0.75	−0.42
5-6 ADLs	2.83	3.34	2.18	−1.16	−0.65
Total	100.00	100.00	100.00	0.00	0.00
Row Percent	100.00	55.87	44.13	−11.74	---

to the 35.6% estimated for age 85 and older in Table 6. The discrepancy declines 6% per 10 years of age with estimates converging at ages 85 to 89.

Table 7 shows the disability distributions observed in 1989; and the age standardized (to the 1989 distribution) disability distribution for the two education groups.

In Table 5, column 4, a difference of 5.73% in disability between the two groups was indicated. After age standardization, the difference was reduced to 4.02% (Table 7, col. 4) because the older population is, on average, less educated than the younger population (Table 6, row per-

TABLE 6: Disability Levels for Noninstitutional Persons Aged 65 Years and Older, by Age and Education–Percent Distribution, United States 1989

Disability Level	(1) Total	(2) Up to High School	(3) High School Graduate	(4) Difference (3)-(2)	(5) Difference (3)-(1)
			Age 65-74 Years		
Nondisabled	89.49	88.33	90.77	2.44	1.28
IADLs	3.13	3.69	2.50	−1.19	−0.63
1-2 ADLs	4.06	4.51	3.55	−0.96	−0.51
3-4 ADLs	1.87	1.81	1.93	0.12	0.06
5-6 ADLs	1.46	1.66	1.25	−0.41	−0.21
Total	100.00	100.00	100.00	0.00	0.00
Row Percent	100.00	52.58	47.42	−5.16	---
			Age 75-84 Years		
Nondisabled	76.09	73.79	79.53	5.74	3.44
IADLs	6.35	7.14	5.17	−1.97	−1.18
1-2 ADLs	9.12	9.86	8.02	−1.84	−1.10
3-4 ADLs	4.89	5.30	4.28	−1.02	−0.61
5-6 ADLs	3.54	3.90	3.00	−0.90	−0.54
Total	100.00	100.00	100.00	0.00	0.00
Row Percent	100.00	59.92	40.08	−19.84	---
			Age 85+ Years		
Nondisabled	48.74	45.54	54.51	8.97	5.77
IADLs	9.13	10.25	7.12	−3.13	−2.01
1-2 ADLs	18.74	19.26	17.79	−1.47	−0.95
3-4 ADLs	12.97	13.20	12.55	−0.65	−0.42
5-6 ADLs	10.42	11.75	8.03	−3.72	−2.39
Total	100.00	100.00	100.00	0.00	0.00
Row Percent	100.00	64.39	35.61	−28.78	---

cents). Thus, 70.2% of the difference of 5.73% was due to education and 29.8% of the difference to the age distribution.

The age-standardized differences in column 5 of Table 7 illustrate what the distribution of disability would be like if all persons had the disability rates of high school graduates. The disabled population is decreased 2.33 percentage points on a base of 17.99%; the relative decline is 13.0%. The high school graduation rate of 82.0% for ages 25 to 64 in 1989 is probably more realistic than the 100% implicit in column 5. If an 82.0% graduation rate is assumed, the weighted average of columns 2 and 3 is 16.38%–1.61 percentage points lower than column 1; the relative decrease is 8.9%. Because of the possible bias, this is an underestimate with the true effect larger. Thus, if these associations hold, and education increases, disability will continue to decline.

Dimensions of Disability

Assessments of long-term care needs frequently use counts of ADL impairments; for example, disability on 2 or more of 5 ADLs, 3 or more of 5 ADLs, or 3 or more of 6 ADLs are considered as thresholds for the need for long-term care. These are readily represented in projection matrices (Table 3). ADL disabilities also tend to be acquired in the order of bathing, dressing, toileting, mobility (bed; other transferring), and eating (Katz & Akpom, 1976). For this reason, linear scales are often used to analyze disability.

TABLE 7: Age Standardized Disability Levels for Noninstitutional Persons Aged 65 Years and Older, by Education–Percent Distribution, United States 1989

Disability Level	(1) Total	(2) Up to High School	(3) High School Graduate	(4) Difference (3)-(2)	(5) Difference (3)-(1)
Nondisabled	82.01	80.32	84.34	4.02	2.33
IADLs	4.63	5.31	3.72	−1.59	−0.91
1-2 ADLs	6.83	7.38	6.09	−1.29	−0.74
3-4 ADLs	3.70	3.82	3.51	−0.31	−0.19
5-6 ADLs	2.83	3.16	2.34	−0.82	−0.49
Total	100.00	100.00	100.00	0.00	0.00

NOTES:
Cols. (2) and (3): Age standardized rates; education and age specific rates applied to total age specific noninstitutional population distribution in 1989.

Linear ADL scales do not fully represent the complex relations of morbidity, disability, and mortality, and between those factors and education, income, and family and social support. Alternately, the basic measures can be analyzed to summarize those relations for projections. Projections are difficult to make without such data reductions because of the large number of parameters. With 6 ADLs, the number of combinations is 26 = 64; with two categories for IADLs and institutionalization, 28 = 256. Thus, the 6 × 6 matrix in Table 3 would be replaced by a 256 × 256 = 65,536 cell matrix. Estimating statistically stable rates for each cell in such a large matrix is difficult. The problem increases exponentially as covariates are added.

There are ways these issues can be resolved. Crucial to the resolution is recognizing the difficulty of treating each disability level as a category. This is not a sensitive way to describe individual differences in multiple dimensions of disability, especially at late ages where some degree of disability is prevalent (Manton, Stallard, Woodbury, & Dowd, 1994). To construct more reliable and sensitive measures of disability, 27 items from the 1982, 1984, and 1989 NLTCS were used to identify dimensions of disability and to construct scores for individuals on each dimension. These measures, being continuous, allowed for better estimates of active life expectancy by allowing "flows" into and out of disability states. The 27 items include ADLs, IADLs, the difficulty in performing physical tasks (e.g., climbing stairs) and visual acuity–a strong predictor of impairment (Marx, Werner, Cohen, Mansfield, & Feldman, 1992; Salive, Guralnick, Glynn, Christen, Wallace, & Ostfeld, 1994).

The number of dimensions was fixed at six after testing models with four, five, six, and seven dimensions. Scores are restricted to the range 0 to 1, with their sums constrained to 1. A score of 1 on a dimension represents an extreme class in the population. In this case, one class was nondisabled, the other five represented various disability profiles. A seventh was assigned a score of 1 for institutional persons, 0 for all others. The power of this procedure is apparent as covariates are added. The addition of 29 medical conditions increased the dimensionality of the solution for noninstitutionalized elderly from six to seven dimensions (Manton, Stallard, Woodbury, & Dowd, 1994). The definitions of the six dimensions here are also refined. The disability scores can be used in projections and calculations of life tables with covariates. The life tables in Table 8 are for four groups formed by combining scores for the seven dimensions.

In Table 8, active life expectancy estimates based both on continuous scores and on homogeneous disability categories are provided. In both cases, monthly transitions to better or worse disability states, and interac-

TABLE 8: Cohort Life Tables and Disability Scores for Males and Females, With and Without Heterogeneity Within Class Eliminated; Estimates for Persons Reaching Age 65 in Mid-1980s

				Percent of Life Expectancy at Age t in Class			
Age t	Model Type[a]	Proportion Surviving to Age t, l_t (percent)	Life Expectancy at Age t, e_t (years)	Little Impairment No Physical and No, or Mild, Cognitive Disability	Moderate Physical Impairment	Heavy Physical Impairment	Extreme Impairment Mod. ADL, Frail, and Institutional
				Males			
65	Continuous State	100.0	15.6	96.3	0.7	0.6	2.4
	Discrete State	100.0	15.4	93.3	0.7	0.6	2.4
75	Continuous State	69.2	10.3	94.0	0.8	1.0	4.3
	Discrete State	69.7	9.8	92.1	1.0	1.3	5.7
85	Continuous State	33.0	6.1	84.7	1.3	2.4	11.6
	Discrete State	32.5	5.3	73.9	2.0	3.7	20.5
95	Continuous State	6.3	3.4	70.1	1.6	5.3	23.0
	Discrete State	4.0	2.3	34.6	2.8	8.6	54.0
				Females			
65	Continuous State	100.0	20.9	95.6	1.0	0.7	2.7
	Discrete State	100.0	20.9	95.6	1.0	0.7	2.7
75	Continuous State	82.6	14.1	91.8	1.3	1.2	5.7
	Discrete State	83.3	14.0	90.1	1.6	1.4	6.8
85	Continuous State	55.2	8.5	76.6	2.2	2.8	18.5
	Discrete State	56.7	8.0	67.9	3.2	3.5	25.4
95	Continuous State	19.5	5.0	57.4	1.9	5.0	35.7
	Discrete State	18.7	4.0	29.4	3.3	6.1	61.2

Source: Data are from the 1982, 1984, and 1989 National Long Term Care Surveys.
[a]In the continuous state model, an individual can belong to more than one class.

tions of disability with mortality, are modeled. In the continuous case, a person can be a member of more than one group with specific disabilities because the scores on each dimension (which can vary from 0 to 1) represent the degree to which a person is described by each of the groups in the solution. In the discrete case, a person can be only in one group; that is, the score on each dimension is 0 or 1. By allowing continuous variation in groups, the analysis may suggest more function is preserved at later ages–because persons can have different intensities of impairment, and partially retain some functions. This is a more precise description of function in the very elderly. Life tables stratified on discrete disability categories are less precise in describing disability since persons must end up in one of the discrete disability states. Furthermore, life tables with discrete categories were abstracted from the continuous state model. To achieve a comparable level of fit, a discrete state model requires more dimensions than a continuous state model.

The age trajectory of monthly changes in function is plotted in Figure 1. These are the projected average monthly scores for nondisabled males and females.

For males, the average monthly decline is 0.090% at ages to 65 to 74; 0.123% at 75 to 84, and 0.115% (or, relatively, 6.5% less) at 85 and older. For females, the monthly decline at ages 65 to 74 is 0.100% or, relatively, 10% more than for males; at 75 to 84, the decline is 0.174, or, relatively, 51% more than for males; and at 85 and older, 0.118 or, relatively, 2.6% more than for males. The declines in the active group score are redistributed to the six disability types. The largest gender difference is the institutional transition which is higher at all ages; and at age 85 and older is, relatively, 169% higher for females. Accounting for the higher institutional rate at age 85 and older, the loss of function for females is half that for males.

At age 90, the decline in function for both genders stops due to the high mortality of severely disabled persons. In the model, declines above age 93 were constrained to be constant. In fact, the average functional status among survivors age 95 and older tends to increase in the population due to mortality selection (Manton, Stallard, Woodbury, & Dowd, 1994). Declines in the mean at age 90 stop because the mortality of the disabled population is roughly the size of the increment due to functional declines of nondisabled survivors. At older ages (e.g., 95 and older), where mortality is higher, the population decline reverses if functional declines for individuals are not sufficient to replace the fraction of the disabled population lost to mortality.

FIGURE 1: Proportion Non-Disabled

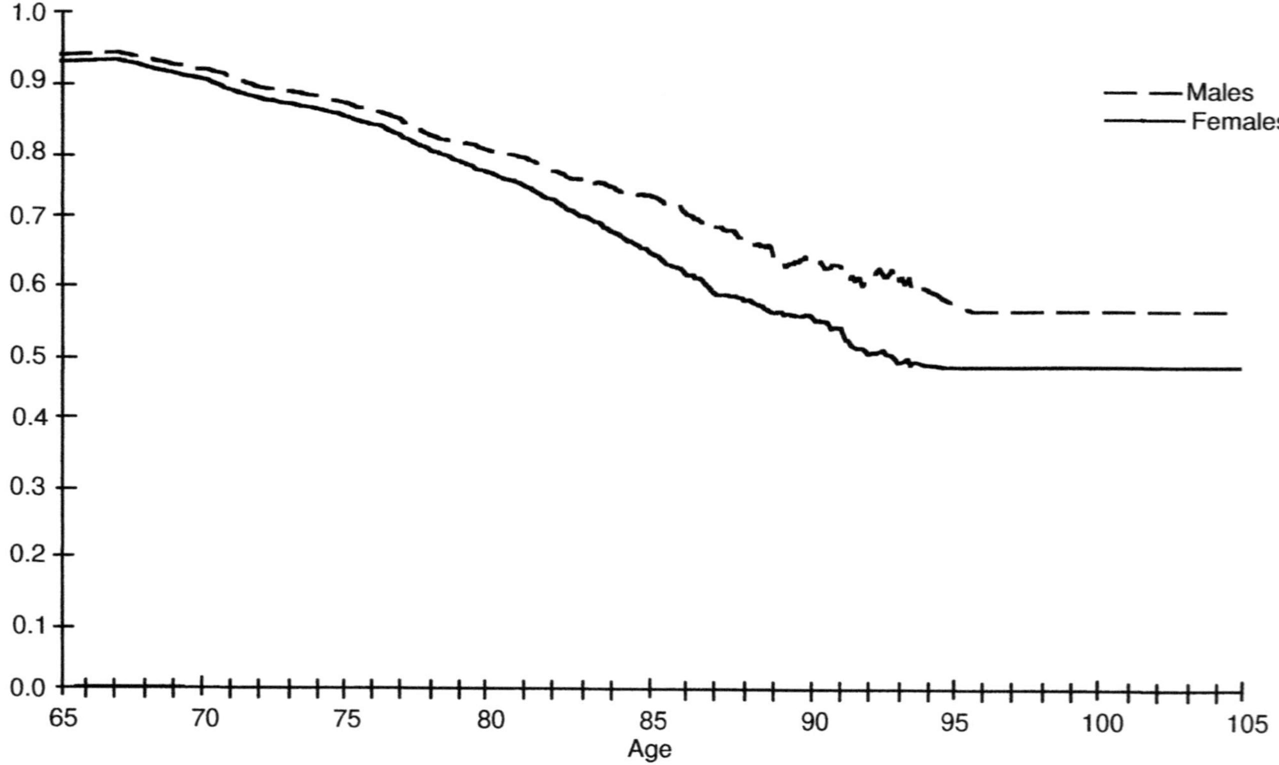

CHANGES IN BIOMEDICAL TECHNOLOGY

Biomedical advances promise to improve function and reduce long-term care costs for the elderly. An evaluation of medical advances suggests that the boundary between acute medical care and new forms of long-term care may become diffuse over time. This study also examined congestive heart failure and the use of angiotensin converting enzyme-II (ACE-II) inhibitors and cardiac pacemakers; the use of exogenous estrogens and the effect on osteoporosis and cardiovascular disease; the effects of surgical procedures on cataracts; the effects of treatments for gastritis and ulcers; and the effects of erythropoietin on the End Stage Renal Disease Program.

Congestive Heart Failure

As treatment improves, the chances of surviving a heart attack, preventing a heart attack in a person with compromised coronary circulation, or of preventing a second heart attack all increase, along with the risk of congestive heart failure. Age-standardized hospitalization rates for congestive heart failure increased by over 60% between 1973 and 1986 (Ghali, Cooper, & Ford, 1990). In contrast to stroke and acute heart disease, congestive heart failure mortality increased up to 1988. Each year, 750,000 cases of congestive heart failure are diagnosed.

Two interventions may reverse these trends. One is the use of cardiac pacemakers. Though pacemakers have been used for a long time (national guidelines were issued in 1984), the sophistication of devices has changed. Currently, 450,000 persons have pacemakers; 85% are over age 65. More than 75,000 pacemakers were implanted in 1988. The ventricular pacemaker (with preset heart rate) improved one- and five-year survival in persons with complete heart block. There have been two major changes in pacemaker technology. One is to make pacing responsive to physiological demand. Variable demand pacemakers improved exercise capacity, functioning, and quality of life in a double blind, randomized crossover study of elderly patients (mean age 75). Second, dual-chamber sequential pacemakers coordinate the pumping of the atrium and ventricle. Atrial contraction accounts for an increasing proportion of ventricular filling with age so that such pacemakers are important for the elderly. Dual chamber sequential pacemakers have both reduced symptoms and increased survival in patients aged 70 and older, over that achieved by older pacemakers; for example, for the "sick sinus" syndrome, five-year mortality declined from 30% to 16%, or by half. Stroke and atrial fibrillation incidence have also declined. In one study of ventricular pacemakers, after seven years of follow-up, mortality declined from 50% to 22% with dual-chamber pacemakers. Another found that dual-chamber pacemakers increased five-year survival rates for congestive heart failure from 57% to 75% (Bush & Finucane, 1994).

New medications have been developed to treat congestive heart failure. ACE-II inhibitors not only control hypertension but may foster remodeling of cardiac muscle such that left ventricular hypertrophy related fibrotic changes are reduced. ACE-II inhibitors reduced, in three years, premature congestive heart failure deaths by 5%, and hospitalizations by 35%. Using conservative estimates, ACE inhibitors' cost efficacy ($9,500 per year of life saved) was two to three times that of standard hypertensive treatment ($25,000 per year of life saved) or for end stage renal disease ($35,000 per year of life saved) (Paul, Kuntz, Eagle, & Weinstein, 1994). National Long Term Care Survey morbidity data (Table 4) did not show declines in all "other" heart diseases due to the recency of ACE-II inhibitor therapy in congestive heart failure. The effects of ACE inhibitors are not restricted to congestive heart failure. They reduce the risk of nephropathy in diabetics (Chan, Cochran, Nicholls, Cheunh, & Swaminathan, 1992). Improved hypertensive treatments have increased the peak age of incidence of renal failure from the fourth to fifth decade of life (Qualheim, Rostand, Kirk, & Luke, 1991).

Exogenous Estrogens

In 1985, three million women took exogenous estrogens to reduce menopausal symptoms. Recently, exogenous estrogens (balanced with progesterones) were shown to reduce both osteoporosis and circulatory disease (Riggs & Melton, 1992; Stampfer, Colditz, Willett, Manson, Rosner, Speizer, & Hennekens, 1991). Not only are exogenous estrogens effective in reducing heart disease, but they also improve risk factor profiles, for example, blood lipids, blood sugar, and so forth (Belchetz, 1994). Estrogens may also affect dementia because much of the dementia over age 85 has a significant circulatory component (Skoog, Nilsson, Palmertz, Andreasson, & Svanborg, 1993). Evidence for such effects is found in data on apolipoprotein E subtypes. E4 is associated with excess Alzheimer's disease risk (Strittmatter, Saunders, Schmechel, Pericak-Vance, Enghild, Salvesen, & Roses, 1993) and cardiovascular disease risk.

Cataract Surgery

Treatment of cataracts has been estimated to cost Medicare $3.2 billion per year (Taylor, 1993). Two lens replacement operations (extracapsular cataract removal with insertion of lens "code 66984" and laser surgery, secondary cataract "code 66821") with combined costs of $2.2 billion represent 20% of all Medicare-allowed surgical charges for physicians (HFCA, 1993). More important are their effects on function. Vision impairment (both cataracts and glaucoma) has been found to reduce functioning in five of seven ADLs in institutionalized patients (Marx, Werner, & Cohen-Mansfield, 1992). Vision impairment has also been related to disability and physical mobility (Salive, Guralnik, Glynn, Christen, Wallace, & Ostfeld, 1994). Thus, better management of vision impairment can affect both function and, by affecting physical activity, chronic disease.

Ulcers and Gastritis

Ulcers and gastritis at late ages are due to many causes including use of nonsteroidal anti-inflammatory drugs and reduced gastric immunity. Recently, it was discovered that most stomach ulcers may be caused by a bacteria, H. pylori. Many gastric ulcers are cured by eradication of H. pylori without anti-acid treatment (e.g., Hosking et al., 1994). This is important since the single most costly drug used to treat gastric ulcers, the anti-acid Zantac, costs $2 billion per year.

End Stage Renal Disease

End stage renal disease is of interest because of the rapid increases in the cost of treatment and high per case costs. Medicare end stage renal disease costs in 1990 were $5.2 billion. Approximately 40.2% of 128,546 dialysis patients (51,596) were over age 65, and 14.1% (18,082) over 75. These were the fastest growing end stage renal disease age groups from 1985 to 1990, increasing annually by 10.0% for those 65 to 74, 15.6% for those 75 and older.

Common causes of end stage renal disease are hypertension (26.5%) and diabetes (25.7%) (HCFA, 1993). Thus, there is potential for prevention (e.g., through ACE-II inhibitors) in 52.2% of cases. A consequence of long-term dialysis is chronic anemia and the physical disability it generates. Since 1988, erythropoietin has been used to treat the effects of anemia, at a cost of $213 million in 1990 (HCFA, 1993).

The population aged 65 and older, though small numerically, is also the fastest growing group in the kidney transplant program (40% per annum increase 1985 to 1990; HCFA, 1993). Thus, with more than 40% of the dialysis population in the End Stage Renal Disease Program now over age 65, the program is becoming oriented to the elderly, a subpopulation for which there are multiple interventions and for which new biomedical technology has a large impact.

New Technologies

Selected biomedical advances have been reviewed here, most of which have only recently become broadly used (and hence, were unlikely to have caused the 1982 to 1989 disability reductions), but which have the potential to further reduce disability–in part, by translating long-term care costs to more acute interventions. We can expect more interventions to emerge (e.g., more joint, knee, and hip replacement surgery to deal with osteoarthritis; improvements in immunological treatment for influenza and pneumonia; better treatment to maintain bone [e.g., salmon calcitonin, diphosphonates]) within five to 10 years. What impact will these interventions have on long-term care needs?

The question also arises as to whether long-term care efficacy can be enhanced by housing interventions and home care. Among chronically disabled persons in 1989, the proportion relying on personal assistance to meet the needs generated by their disability declined while the proportion using special equipment and housing to meet needs increased (Manton, Corder, & Stallard, 1993b). In 1982, 314,000 disabled persons used only special equipment to cope with disability (6.5% of the total disabled). By 1989, this increased to 631,000 (12%), a relative increase of 101.2%. The number using only assistance declined from 1,509,000 in 1982 (31.2%) to 1,118,000 (21.2%) in 1989–a relative decline of 25.9%. The number of persons using both equipment and assistance increased from 2,940,000 (60.7%) to 3,436,000 (65.1%), a relative increase of 16.9%. Thus, there is increased reliance on equipment in managing disability, which might increase long-term care cost effectiveness.

In long-term care demonstrations, specific groups could be identified, for whom community services were more effective. In the Channeling[1] data this group contained better-educated females–even without extensive housing and social resources (Manton, Vertrees, & Clark, 1993). The efficacy of services is determined by the development of screening to better diagnose problems in elderly patients with multiple conditions. One effective intervention is the geriatric evaluation and management unit. A problem with such units is the lack of geriatricians. The Veterans Administration has increased geriatric evaluation and management unit use in its hospitals. Those that are appropriately staffed discharge more persons home (63.4% vs. 40.0%), fewer persons to nursing homes (19.1% vs.

40.3%), and after a shorter length of stay (25.4 days vs. 69.9 days) (Wieland, Lubenstein, Hedrick, Rubens, & Buchner, 1994).

CHANGES IN THE DELIVERY OF POST-ACUTE SERVICES BY MEDICARE

Changes in Medicare service use may meet, in part, the projected long-term care need. In 1981, restrictions on the number of home health agency (HHA) visits were lifted. In 1983, Medicare reimbursement of short stay hospitals was shifted to the Prospective Payment System (PPS). Restraint on the growth of physician payments under Medicare Supplemental Medical Insurance was accomplished by the Deficit Reduction Act of 1984, which froze payments for 15 months, starting in July 1984. This was extended by Congress to April 1986 (or December 1986, depending on whether the physician participated in the program or not). More comprehensive controls of physician fees were mandated by the Omnibus Budget Reconciliation Act of 1989, beginning in January 1, 1992, with a five-year phase-in of a fee schedule based on relative value costs for 7,000 services. The Department of Health and Human Services has mandated research on a PPS-type system suitable for bundling charges for outpatient services.

It was thought that PPS-shortened hospital stays and reduced hospitalization rates might stimulate skilled nursing facility (SNF) and HHA use. Increases did not initially materialize. General Accounting Office and internal Health Care Financing Administration studies criticized management of the HHA benefit (HCFA, 1993) causing denial rates to more than double by 1987. Instead, outpatient service use grew manifold between 1983 and 1990.

In 1988, the Duggan vs. Bowen suit was settled, revising the definition of intermittent care. This was promulgated in the regulations introduced by HCFA in mid-1989. In 1988, the Medicare Catastrophic Care Act was passed. Repealed in 1989, it is viewed as little affecting Medicare use. However, it liberalized benefits in ways that caused nursing home proprietors to upgrade facilities to become Medicare-eligible. OBRA 1987 required Medicaid facilities to be Medicare certifiable. Consequently, 1,624 SNFs were created with 75,000 beds–many in underserved areas.

The consequences of these developments are shown in Table 9.

Both SNF and HHA use changed from 1982 to 1989; for example, the number using HHA increased from 1.31 to 1.86 million persons. The number of visits increased from 36 to 72 million per year. The number of

TABLE 9: Annual Use of HHA and SNF Services in 1982-1983 and 1989-1990 for Persons Aged 65 Years and Older, by Disability Level, United States

	HHA USE				SNF USE		
Disability Level	(1) Observed 1982-1983	(2) Observed 1989-1990	(3) Expected 1989-1990	Disability Level	(1) Observed 1982-1983	(2) Observed 1989-1990	(3) Expected 1989-1990
NON-DISABLED				NON-DISABLED			
Visits/Enrollee	0.62	1.22		SNF Days/Enrollee	0.14	0.28	
Percent Using Services	2.95%	3.95%		Percent Using Services	0.45%	0.86%	
Average Visits/User	21.2	30.8		Average Days/User	30.7	32.4	
Total HHA visits (000's)	12,447	28,148	14,339	Total SNF Days (000's)	2,721	6,463	3,238
Persons Using Services (000's)	587	914	682	Persons Using Services (000's)	88	200	104
IADL ONLY				IADL ONLY			
Visits/Enrollee	1.67	4.45		SNF Days/Enrollee	0.41	0.97	
Percent Using Services	6.79%	11.81%		Percent Using Services	1.25%	2.04%	
Average Visits/User	24.6	37.7		Average Days/User	32.8	47.9	
Total HHA Visits (000's)	2,322	5,853	2,197	Total SNF Days (000's)	569	1,283	540
Persons Using Services (000's)	94,442	155	89	Persons Using Services (000's)	17	27	16
I-2 ADL				1-2 ADL			
Visits/Enrollee	3.39	4.86		SNF Days/Enrollee	0.71	1.65	
Percent Using Services	12.81%	14.32%		Percent Using Services	2.14%	4.97%	
Average Visits/User	26.5	34.0		Average Days/User	33.0	33.1	
Total HHA Visits (000's)	5,719	9,379	6,538	Total SNF Days (000's)	1,192	3,176	1,369
Persons Using Services (000's)	216	276	246	Persons Using Services (000's)	36	96	41

3-4 ADL			
Visits/Enrollee	7.02	9.71	
Percent Using Services	19.61%	23.66%	
Average Visits/User	35.8	41.1	
Total HHA Visits (000's)	4,986	10,142	7,329
Persons Using Services (000's)	139	247	204
5-6 ADL			
Visits/Enrollee	10.7	21.06	
Percent Using Services	25.76%	29.05%	
Average Visits/User	41.6	72.5	
Total HHA Visits (000's)	9,750	17,288	8,783
Persons Using Services (000's)	234	238	211
INSTITUTIONAL			
Visits/Enrollee	0.61	0.81	
Percent Using Services	2.36%	1.82%	
Average Visits/User	25.8	44.6	
Total HHA Visits (000's)	904	1,321	994
Persons Using Services (000's)	35	29	38
TOTAL			
Visits/Enrollee	1.38	2.42	
Percent Using Services	5.01%	6.23%	
Average Visits/User	27.6	38.8	
Total HHA Visits (000's)	36,130	72,133	41,218
Persons Using Services (000's)	1,307	1,860	1,496

3-4 ADL			
SNF Days/Enrollee	0.62	2.00	
Percent Using Services	2.29%	6.67%	
Average Days/User	27.2	30.0	
Total SNF Days (000's)	441	2,090	647
Persons Using Services (000's)	16	70	24
5-6 ADL			
SNF Days/Enrollee	1.35	2.79	
Percent Using Services	4.11%	6.85%	
Average Days/User	32.9	40.8	
Total SNF Days (000's)	1,229	2,292	1,108
Persons Using Services (000's)	37	56	34
INSTITUTIONAL			
SNF Days/Enrollee	1.2	6.03	
Percent Using Services	3.51%	10.03%	
Average Days/User	34.1	60.1	
Total SNF Days (000's)	1,779	9,834	1,956
Persons Using Services (000's)	52	163	57
TOTAL			
SNF Days/Enrollee	0.3	0.84	
Percent Using Services	0.95%	2.05%	
Average Days/User	32.0	41.1	
Total SNF Days (000's)	7,933	25,139	8,960
Persons Using Services (000's)	248	612	284

NOTES: Col. (3)– Based on 1982-1983 rates.
Source: Tabulations of HHA and SNF use for the 1982 and 1989 NLTCS sample population prepared by the Center for Demographic Studies, Duke University

visits per user increased from roughly 28 to 39. The proportion of the Medicare elderly population using HHA increased from 5.01% to 6.23%.

SNFs changes were equally large. From 248,000 persons using SNFs for 12 months after the end of the survey in October 1982, use expanded to 612,000 persons using services in the 12 months after the end of the survey in October 1989. The number of SNF days per user increased from 32.0 to 41.1 days (from 7.9 to 25.1 million SNF days per year). Costs increased for HHA from $1.8 billion (in 1990 dollars) per year in 1982 to 1983 to $3.8 billion in 1989 to 1990. SNF costs increased from $441 million per year in 1982 to 1983 to $2.2 billion per year in 1989 to 1990. Thus, for 1989 to 1990, Medicare HHA and SNF costs were $6.0 billion. Increases are not equally distributed over disability level. The number of HHA visits used by those with five to six ADLs almost doubled from 9.8 to 17.3 million per year. The number of SNF days used by those in institutions increased over five-fold from 1.8 to 9.8 million per year. SNF use rose more rapidly for the more disabled population while HHA use increased more, relatively, for less disabled populations.

HHA visits grew from 47 million in 1989 to 70 million in 1990 (+49%), and to 98 million in 1991 (+40%) (HCFA, 1993). SNF days used increased 140% from 1988 to 1989. The trends for all Medicare HHA and SNF costs for 1989 to 1992 are in Table 10.

By 1992, SNF and HHA costs increased to $10.9 billion. By 1994, the figure might be $18 billion. Without controls, HHA use could be 10% of Medicare costs by 2000. Given the differential use of HHA and SNF services across disability levels, and the increased use of both services (Table 9), the growth of SNF use (from 1988 to 1989 and in 1992) and HHA use (from 1989 on) has significantly affected long-term care needs.

Finally, there is the issue of the degree to which acute and long-term care costs are substitutable. Should costs for other Medicare services be viewed as contributing to long-term care needs (e.g., cataract surgery)? If so, should the effects of such procedures on long-term care costs be counted because they reduce long-term care needs below those expected in the absence of such procedures?

CONCLUSION

This article has reviewed data on changes in the U.S. elderly population, its service use, and implications of those changes for long-term care. Difficult issues are raised concerning the forecasting of a complex array of related processes. Because of the difficulty in addressing these issues, and

TABLE 10: Medicare Expenditures in $Millions, by Type of Service and Calendar Year 1989 to 1992, United States

Type of Service	1989	1990	1991	1992
Inpatient Hospital	53,822	59,301	63,167	69,007
% Change		+10.2%	+6.5%	+9.2%
Outpatient Hospital	7,662	8,475	9,756	10,671
% Change		+10.6%	+15.1%	+9.4%
Physician	27,057	29,628	32,231	32,304
% Change		+9.5%	+8.8%	+0.2%
Group Practice	2,308	2,827	3,524	3,810
% Change		+22.5%	+24.7%	+8.1%
SNF	2,978	2,876	2,520	3,692
% Change		−3.4%	−12.4%	+46.5%
HHA	2,838	3,598	5,200	7,162
% Change		+26.8%	+44.5%	+37.7%

Source: National Center for Health Statistics. Health, United States, 1993; p. 243, 1994.

the likely costs of a solution, no U.S. long-term care policy has yet been implemented.

Initial costs for proposed long-term care programs are in the $40 billion range. Variation in initial costs, and their rate of growth are of concern. These problems might be dealt with by capping both the initial program size and the growth rate. But while this would remove uncertainty, it would not solve problems in assessing and forecasting the array of processes determining true long-term care needs. Required is a review of basic strategies and the promotion of emerging positive health trends through targeted funding mechanisms. In this way, it may be possible to deal with a larger proportion of the total long-term care problem than we are now dealing with, and to identify what parts and how much of the problem remain to be solved and what new and old solutions should be considered.

ENDNOTE

1. The National Channeling Demonstration was a large study conducted by the Assistant Secretary's Office for Policy and Evaluation of the use of case management services in directing disabled persons towards different types of community

long-term care services. The demonstration took place in 10 sites and followed persons for approximately 18 months. In one area of the study, case management was combined with supplementary benefits.

REFERENCES

Belchetz, P.E. (1994). Hormonal treatment of postmenopausal women. *New England Journal of Medicine*, *330*(15), 1062-1071.

Bush, D.E., & Finucane, T.E. (1994). Permanent cardiac pacemakers in the elderly. *Journal of the American Geriatrics Society*, *42*, 326-334.

Chan, J., Cockram, C., Nicholls, M., Cheunh, C. & Swaminathan, R. (1992). Comparison of enalapril and nifedipine in treating non-insulin dependent diabetes associated with hypertension: One year analysis. *British Medical Journal*, *305*, 981-985.

Evans, D.A., Scherr, P.A., Cook, N.R. et al. (1992). The impact of Alzheimer's disease in the United States population. In K. Manton, B. Singer, & R. Suzman (Eds.), *Forecasting the health of elderly populations* (pp. 283-299). New York: Springer-Verlag.

Fogel, Robert W. (1993). Economic growth, population theory, and physiology: The bearing of long-term processes on the making of economic policy. *The American Economic Review*, *84*(3), 369-395.

Ghali, J.K., Cooper, R., & Ford, E. (1990). Trends in hospitalization rates for heart failure in the United States, 1973-1986. *Archives of Internal Medicine*, *150*, 769-776.

Hannan, M. T., Anderson, J. J., Pincus, T., & Felson, D.T. (1992). Educational attainment and osteoarthritis: Differential associations with radiographics changes and symptom reporting. *Journal of Clinical Epidemiology*, *45*(2), 139-147.

Health Care Financing Administration. (1993). *Health Care Financing Review*, Medicare and Medicaid Statistical Supplement (Annual Supplement). Baltimore, MD: U.S. Government Printing Office.

Hosking, S., Ling, T., Chung, S., Yung, M., Cheng, A., Sung, J., & Li, A. (1994). Duodenal ulcer healing by eradication of helicobacter pylori without anti-acid treatment: Randomized controlled trial. *The Lancet*, *343*, 508-510.

Katz, S., & Akpom, C. (1976). A measure of primary sociobiological functions. *International Journal of Health Services*, *6*, 493-508.

Lanska, D.J., & Mi, X. (1993). Decline in U.S. stroke mortality in the era before antihypertensive therapy. *Stroke*, *24*(9), 1382-1388.

Lawton, M.P., & Brody, E.M. (1969). Assessment of older people: Self-maintaining and instrumental activities of daily living. *The Gerontologist*, *2*, 179-186.

Manton, K.G., Corder, L.S., & Stallard, E. (1993a). Estimates of change in chronic disability and institutional incidence and prevalence rates in the U.S. elderly population from the 1982, 1984, and 1989 National Long Term Care Survey. *Journal of Gerontology: Social Sciences*, *47*(4), S153-S166.

Manton, K.G., Corder, L.S., & Stallard E. (1993b). Changes in the use of personal assistance and special equipment 1982 to 1989: Results from the 1982 and 1989 NLTCS. *The Gerontologist, 33*, 168-176.
Manton, K.G., Stallard, E., & Corder, L.S. (1995). Changes in morbidity and chronic disability in the U.S. elderly population: Evidence from the 1982, 1984, and 1989 National Long Term Care Surveys. *Journal of Gerontology: Social Services, 50*(4), S194-S204.
Manton, K.G., Stallard, E., Woodbury, M.A., & Dowd, J.E. (1994). Time varying covariates of human mortality and aging: Multidimensional generalizations of the Gompertz. *Journal of Gerontology: Biological Sciences, 49*, B169-B190.
Manton, K.G., Vertrees, J.C., & Clark, R.F. (1993). A multivariate analysis of disability and health and its change over time in the National Channeling Demonstration data. *The Gerontologist, 33*(5), 610-618.
Marx, M.S., Werner, P., Cohen-Mansfield, J., & Feldman, R. (1992). The relationship between low vision and performance of activities of daily living in nursing home residents. *Journal of the American Geriatrics Society, 40*(10), 1018-1020.
Mozar, H.N., Bal, D.G., & Farag, S.A. (1990). The natural history of atherosclerosis: An ecologic perspective. *Atherosclerosis, 82*, 157-164.
National Center for Health Statistics. (1994). *Health. United States. 1993*. Hyattsville, MD: Public Health Service.
Paul, S.D., Kuntz, K.M., Eagle, K.A., & Weinstein, M.C. (1994). Costs and effectiveness of angiotensin converting enzyme inhibitors in patients with congestive heart failure. *Archives of Internal Medicine, 154*, 1143-1149.
Preston, S.H. (1992). Demographic change in the United States, 1970-2050. In K. Manton, B. Singer, & R. Suzman (Eds.), *Forecasting the health of elderly populations* (pp. 51-78). New York: Springer-Verlag.
Qualheim, R.E., Rostand, S.G., Kirk, K.A., & Luke, R.G. (1991). Changing patterns of end-stage renal disease due to hypertension. *American Journal of Kidney Disease, 18*, 336-343.
Riggs, B., & Melton, I.L. (1992). Drug therapy: The prevention and treatment of osteoporosis. *New England Journal of Medicine, 327*(9), 620-627.
Salive, M.E., Guralnik, J., Glynn, R.J., Christen, W., Wallace, R.B., & Ostfeld, A.M. (1994). Association of visual impairment with mobility and physical function. *Journal of the American Geriatrics Society, 42*, 287-292.
Skoog, I., Nilsson, L., Palmertz, B., Andreasson, L.A., & Svanborg, A. (1993). A population-based study of dementia in 85-year-olds. *New England Journal of Medicine, 328*(3), 153-158.
Stampfer, M.J., Colditz, G.A., Willett, W.C., Manson, J.E., Rosner, B., Speizer, F.E., & Hennekens, C.H. (1991). Postmenopausal estrogen therapy and cardiovascular disease: Ten-year follow-up from the nurses health study. *New England Journal of Medicine, 325*, 756-762.
Strittmatter, J.W., Saudners, A.M., Schmechel, D., Pericak-Vance, M., Enghild, J., Salvesen, G.S., & Roses, A. (1993). Apolipoprotein E: High-avidity binding to

b-amyloid and increased frequency of type 4 allele in late-onset familial Alzheimer's disease. *Proceedings of the National Academy of Sciences*, *90*, 1977-1981.

Taylor, A. (1993). Cataract: Relationships between nutrition and oxidation. *Journal of the American College of Nutrition*, *12*(2), 138-146.

U.S. Bureau of the Census. (1992). Current Population Reports, Special Studies, P23-178, *Sixty-five plus in America*. Washington, DC: U.S. Government Printing Office.

Wieland, D., Rubenstein, L.Z., Hedrick, S.C., Reuben, D.B., & Buchner, D.M. (1994). Inpatient geriatric evaluation and management units (GEMs) in the Veterans health system: Diamonds in the rough. *Journal of Gerontology: Medical Sciences*, *49*(5), M195-M200.

ACCESS VS. NEED IN LONG-TERM CARE TODAY

Home and Community-Based Care: Recent Accomplishments and New Challenges

Robert B. Hudson, PhD

Boston University School of Social Work
Boston, Massachusetts

SUMMARY. This article traces the development of home and community-based care to its current place in the worlds of health and social policy. An argument is developed to the effect that such services have by now gained both heightened policy legitimacy and organiza-

Robert B. Hudson is Professor and Chair, Department of Social Welfare Policy, Boston University School of Social Work. He has written widely on aging policy issues and serves as Editor of *The Public Policy and Aging Report,* the publication of the National Academy on Aging.

Dr. Hudson can be contacted at Boston University's School of Social Work, 264 Bay State Road, Boston, MA 02215.

[Haworth co-indexing entry note]: "Home and Community-Based Care: Recent Accomplishments and New Challenges." Hudson, Robert B. Co-published simultaneously in *Journal of Aging & Social Policy* (The Haworth Press, Inc.) Vol. 7, No. 3/4, 1996, pp. 53-69; and: *From Nursing Homes to Home Care* (ed: Marie E. Cowart and Jill Quadagno) The Haworth Press, Inc., 1996, pp. 53-69. Single or multiple copies of this article are available from The Haworth Document Delivery Service [1-800-342-9678, 9:00 a.m. - 5:00 p.m. (EST)].

tional capacity. Building on these contentions, the article goes on to suggest that such services should continue to gain a more prominent place within long-term care policy, and that long-term care issues deserve a more central place within social insurance policy more generally. The article concludes by suggesting that demonstrations of policy efficacy such as those that are taking place in home and community services might help to at least modestly offset the frontal assault which is currently taking place across the range of American social policy. *[Article copies available from The Haworth Document Delivery Service: 1-800-342-9678.]*

The emergence of home and community-based long-term care services in the United States has been a major development in the heretofore largely discrete worlds of health care and social service provision. Until roughly the mid-1970s, long-term care was understood to be almost entirely institutionally based, whether in an almshouse, a state facility, a rehabilitation hospital, or a nursing home. Until only a short time later, "community-based care" referred to social services that facilitated the lives of persons living at home and assisted them in enjoying a variety of services and functions in the larger community. The coming together of *functionally oriented* and *targeted* services designed to keep frail and disabled persons at home who otherwise would be somewhere else is a major conceptual milestone (if still only a small roadside marker in expenditure terms) in health and social service delivery.

This article, first, traces the evolution of home and community-based care to its current place in the worlds of health and social policy, arguing that it has attained a new and needed legitimacy in policy circles. Second, the article documents the heightened system capacity now associated with home and community-based care operations in many parts of the country. The third section suggests reasons why home and community-based care should attain yet greater standing in the policy world, speculating that home and community-based care's broad legitimacy and high potential might serve to breathe some modest level of support for public-sector activity back into today's political discourse.

THE LEGITIMATION OF HOME AND COMMUNITY-BASED CARE

Today's publicly supported home and community-based services in the United States have emerged from two discrete service arenas: the first, centered on the provision of home care services, and the second, incorporating community-based social services.

Home Care for the Chronically Ill and Post-Acute

Key elements in the emergence of home care policy include the disjunctures between health care and welfare programming, the appropriateness and costs of home care as an alternative to both hospital and nursing home care, and the respective roles of social insurance protections and public welfare assistance. The distinction between "medical post-acute" and "social supportive" home care services made by A. E. Benjamin (1993) is helpful in harnessing these convoluted developments as the following discussion demonstrates.

The health and welfare separation dates to the turn of the century and was marked by an early divide between home health services and homemaker services. The former began as nursing services, with the nurses being employed by private visiting-nurse agencies and later by public health departments (Mundlinger, 1983). Homemaker services were developed by charitable agencies and were designed to remove or keep families off of public relief rolls.

This distinction held as policy attention turned increasingly to the old, where community-based service alternatives were part of a long-term and disjointed strategy to keep poor and chronically ill elders out of penury and out of institutions. Concern on the part of reformers and others that the aged poor were largely confined to "indoor relief" settings, which was in fact historically inaccurate (Haber, 1993), led to interest in home care services as alternatives to residency in almshouses or state hospitals. Belief that impoverished elders should be able to maintain themselves in the community was enshrined in the Old Age Assistance (OAA) title of the 1935 Social Security Act, in which OAA cash grants could not be made to "any inmate of a public institution." It was the combination of OAA cash grants, prohibitions on institutional care, and growing levels of frailty among the poor old that led to the subsequent growth of the nursing home industry (Vladeck, 1980).

Later debates surrounding the passage of Medicare and Medicaid continued this post-acute and supportive-service distinction. The home care provisions of the 1965 Medicare and Medicaid legislation further institutionalized this dual home care history. Medicare emphasized post-acute skilled care on an intermittent basis to homebound individuals, with supportive services only incidental to skilled care. In contrast, Medicaid promoted preventive, skilled, and nonskilled care to low-income, chronically ill individuals, and included no prior hospitalization or homebound requirements (Benjamin, 1993).

While legislatively furthering the divide between post-acute and supportive home care services, Medicare and Medicaid also helped set in motion events that would significantly lessen the residual and marginal place of home and community-based care services. Most important was the rise in health care expenditures that occurred subsequent to enactment of the two laws. As a means of stemming the overall expenditure increases, attention slowly focused on nonhospital and nonnursing home alternatives. Thus, between 1967 and 1985, Medicare home health expenditures rose from $43 million to $2.3 billion, and Medicaid home care expenditures rose from $24 million to $1.1 billion (Kavesh, 1986).

Cost concerns have continued to be central to home and community-based care expansion. Post-acute care expenditures have been the primary worry in Washington, both of the Social Security Administration and its health care successor, the Health Care Financing Administration. The states saw escalating Medicaid costs and an expanding portion of those costs attributable to elderly nursing home residents. By the 1980s, the so-called Medicaid 2176 waiver programs and state-only funds were being used with the intent of containing costs and providing appropriate care.

With the formation of the Pepper Commission, the introduction of home care initiatives by Senators Edward M. Kennedy (D-MA), Robert Kerrey (D-NE), Bob Packwood (R-OR), Robert Dole (R-KS), George Mitchell (D-ME), and Rep. Pete Stark (D-CA) in the early 1990s and, of course, President Clinton's later health care reform initiative, home care took a more central place on the health and welfare stage than ever before. The clouded future of home and community-based care and the attendant social policies in light of the Republication revolution in the post-1994 Congress is the topic of this article's concluding section.

SOCIAL SERVICES FOR THE AGED

A second home and community-based care services antecedent is found in the history of voluntarism, mutual aid, and charitable activity in grassroots America (Lubove, 1968), and is based on the "qualities of community" in these nonprofit groups: self-identifying membership, voluntary action, and activities based on deeply held values and shared sentiments (Smith & Lipsky, 1993). Early activities of this type were slowly consolidated into "community chests" and health and welfare councils in the pre-World War II period, but they long continued as indigenous community activities.

Government funding and regulation of these activities related to community services for the old came with enactment of the Older Americans Act in 1965. As a political adjunct to Medicare, the OAA indulged a number of nonmedical political interests (Binstock, 1972); as part of the New Frontier/Great Society "services strategy," it brought to the old community-based supports analogous to job training for the unskilled (Sundquist, 1968) and services for public assistance recipients "to strengthen family life" (Derthick, 1975).

Although, today, activity under the OAA is increasingly directed at the long-term care needs of frail elders, activities under the Act were directed quite differently during its first 20 years. The legislation's first five years were marked by simply establishing designated agencies in each of the states, and in doling out minuscule grants to local community groups. In the subsequent 15 years or so, the OAA took on greater prominence as appropriations skyrocketed from $20 million in 1971 to $212 million in 1973, and to $951 million by 1981. Yet during this period of great expansion (expansion has subsequently leveled off and more recently declined slightly in constant dollar spending), questions about program mission and service eligibility were only marginally focused on those elders most in need of home and community-based care services.

Major debates about matters of service eligibility surfaced by the mid-1970s. The question was no less fundamental than this: Which elders, in fact, was the OAA designed to serve? A cornerstone provision of the law since 1965 was that all persons aged 60 and older were formally entitled to services under the Act. But, during the 1970s, pressures were building on lawmakers and the Administration on Aging to pay greater attention to particular subsets of elders whose needs could be argued to be relatively greater than those of the older population as a whole.

The resultant targeting centered initially on economic and ascriptive population characteristics rather than on illness or impairment. The competing criteria (and the years of the particular amendments) included: low income (1973); greatest social and economic need (1978); low-income minority populations (1984); and low-income minority, rural, and non-English speaking populations (1987) (O'Shaughnessy, 1991). In the absence of means-testing or other quantifiable mandates, implementation of these requirements has proven highly uneven. As a question of both organizational mission and client eligibility, the issue of frailty and functional impairment gradually entered the OAA policy debate beginning in the late-1970s. Robert Benedict, the Commissioner on Aging during the Carter years, declared community-based long-term care services to be a priority activity; he had the social services title–

long a near-laundry list of discrete service activities–sharpened to emphasize activity in three areas: access services, in-home services, and legal services. Of the three service clusters, access and legal services were not nearly so central to clients with impairments as were in-home services. That service emphasis across the country gradually shifted in this last direction is useful in highlighting the transition that began during this period toward emphasizing home-based services under the OAA. This subtle but important shift in purpose was a shift *away* from emphasizing the role of services in assisting elders at home to have access to the community and interesting things to do when they got home *toward* one stressing the development of home and community-based services aimed at allowing frail elders to remain in their own homes, rather than be placed in institutional settings.

Moving toward the present in this historical account, we see an increase among the traditional aging agencies in both the volume and the focus of home and community-based care activity. In 1987, language was added to the OAA that requires states to reach out to elders with disabilities, and in 1989, the Declaration of Objectives under Title I was expanded to include the establishment of community-based long-term care services. In the wake of these legislative changes and home and community-based care policy activity at the state level, roughly one half of OAA appropriations today support home and community-based care.

In the 1980s and 1990s, these historical strands of long-term care policy began to come together. Home and community-based care is no longer a collection of the unintegrated residual elements of health policy, public assistance, and community philanthropy. For the chronically ill poor, long-term care no longer connotes definitionally extended residence in a nursing home or other long-stay institution. For those with acute conditions, home-based and "sub-acute" care are rapidly growing alternatives to hospitalization. And, the activities from the traditional social service worlds such as adult day care and respite care are much more heavily directed toward frail elders than ever before.

The argument to this point is to suggest that, for the reasons enumerated, home and community-based care has today attained a status where it is not solely residual, that is, an alternative to something else. Attaining that status markedly elevates the legitimacy of home and community-based care as a policy option in health and social care. That point established, attention now turns to the question of policy capacity.

THE BUREAUCRATIZATION OF HOME AND COMMUNITY-BASED CARE

These developments have brought greater formalization and heightened capacity to home and community-based care service systems. Most central have been: (a) important shifts in understanding the composition and needs of older and impaired populations in relation to community-based long-term care; and (b) significant refinements in the design and development of home and community-based service systems targeted to those needs. The advent of these client and system-level advances bode well for future home and community-based care programming.

Age, Disability, and Community-Based Care

Contributing to the greater centrality of home and community-based care options for the frail old has been a growing convergence in terms of policy about who home and community-based programs should be serving. Whereas the OAA's traditional concern has been with *client inclusiveness*, Medicaid's has focused on *service intensity*. However, the most recent period has seen a softening in that distinction. Targeting of services under the OAA is increasingly directed toward the functionally impaired, and the states–using Medicaid authorizations and waivers and state-only funding–have broadened the menu of home and community-based care benefits available to impaired populations.

While OAA activity was centered on better concentrating limited dollars, Medicaid home and community-based care activity was directed first on containing nursing home costs and, then, on limiting the volume of demand that might be expected for more popular community-based care alternatives. The need to do both became clear by the early 1990s. Medicaid home health costs were growing rapidly in both absolute and relative terms, while Medicaid nursing home expenditures were also continuing to grow even as such spending came to constitute a slowly declining proportion of overall long-term care spending (U.S. GAO, 1994).

Toward both containing costs and promoting equity, client assessment instruments are now almost universally employed in state-level home and community-based care programs, now including many OAA-based initiatives (Kane, Urv-Wong, & King, 1990). While unquestionably promoting equitable treatment where they are appropriately used, all such instruments leave open questions about what impairments to measure, what measures to use, and how stringently to use them. Though Activities of Daily Living and allied scales are arcane to the uninitiated, they have enormous practice implications. Walter Leutz, Ruby Abrahams, and John

Capitman (1993) note that limiting services to those individuals with only two or three ADL limitations would "define a population of unprecedented narrowness" (p. 94), and Robyn Stone and Daniel Murtaugh (1990) report that eligibility among elders under such limitations might range from 411,000 to 4.1 million persons, depending on how restrictive or expansive the ADL/IADL limits imposed are.

This gradual melding of gatekeeping functions and services is a major development in the context of public policy for the aged. Community-based policy directed at functionally impaired individuals of all ages is moving forward more quickly than most analysts would have anticipated and than recent experience, in fact, suggests (Torres-Gil & Pynoos, 1986). This convergence speaks to greater political activism on the part of younger disabled populations and to a shifting policy perception of who the aged actually are. For the aged, the lesson is clearly that service availability will increasingly be based on demonstrable rather than presumed needs. On its face, that is a fair standard; left unresolved, however, in addition to questions of need and measurement, are the ability and the responsibility for society's meeting demonstrable needs in a manner that reasonably addresses concerns of universality, adequacy, and equity.

Public-Sector Roles and Capacity in Community-Based Care

Closely tied to rationalization of client eligibility criteria has been increasing formalization of the home and community-based care service delivery system. Steps taken in this direction include broadened and intensified use of case management interventions, greater organizational consolidation, and the emergence of state-level agencies as key players in home and community-based care service delivery with a roughly parallel reduction in the federal government's organizational oversight and presence in the delivery of community-based services.

Case management has had a growing place in community-based efforts dating back to the pioneering efforts of the Wisconsin Community Care Organization strategies of the early 1970s. Through the Channeling Demonstration project and the ongoing Medicaid 2176 waiver programs, case management has become a central feature of virtually all home and community-based care efforts. As well, states and communities are introducing increasingly sophisticated and far-reaching case management systems. Rosalie A. Kane and colleagues (1991) extrapolate five models of case management practice from recent experience: broker model, purchase of authority public funds model, managed-care model, private long-term care insurance model, and fee-for-service model.

In her assessment of home and community-based care innovations in six states, Diane Justice (1988) speaks of a consolidated model, in which community and institutional services are integrated into a single purpose agency; an umbrella model, with heightened interdivisional shifting of responsibilities; and a more traditional model, in which separate agencies work together on a formal basis to better coordinate their efforts. Writing from the vantage point of the state agencies, Daniel Quirk (1991) cites home and community-based care advances in five areas: the development of single-client entry points into the system, a growing use of state revenues, the development of nonmedical support services, a greater recognition of the relationship between formal and informal care provision, and the targeting of benefits to persons who meet formally designated impairment criteria.

These developments have led to a marked broadening of responsibility for the state units on aging (SUAs). In a remarkable advance in less than a 10-year period, state units on aging now administer or share in the administration of home and community-based care programs in 38 states, and SUAs administer at least one program beyond the OAA in 42 states (U.S. GAO, 1991). Symbolically, this shift has seen the names of many state agencies change to include, most usually, references to the disabled adult population.

While these developments have brought notable improvements in community-based service delivery for impaired persons, there remain tensions and unresolved questions between home and community-based care delivery networks and traditional social service providers. Richard Fortinksy (1991, p. 4) speaks to the difficulties many aging network agencies have experienced in the "shift in the priority from social and recreational services to personal care and household assistance services, from emphasis on social and economic needs to health and functional needs." Catherine Alter (1988) documents such tensions in her comparison of two county-based systems, one large and sprawling but relatively autonomous and involving of nonprofessional personnel, and the other much more highly bureaucratized and efficient, but subject to morale problems associated with highly formalized structures.

My review of capacity-building activity in four Area Agencies on Aging of Alter's first type found these small agencies relying heavily on the OAA Title III congregate nutrition program to support other community-oriented activities (Hudson, 1983). This finding is instructive in that recent amendments (and pending "aging block-grant" proposals) authorize the transferring of congregate nutrition funds to in-home nutrition services. That the transfers are moving toward in-home meal provision and away from congregate provision suggests that the service offerings of the more traditional community agencies, whatever their merits, are a vanishing commodity in publicly supported service systems. Indeed, they are likely to disappear altogether unless they are resurrected under some other local auspice.

THE CASE FOR EXPANDED PUBLIC-SECTOR LONG-TERM CARE EFFORTS

The essence of my argument to this point has been that we have seen remarkable progress in the development of home and community-based care systems along two critical policy dimensions: legitimacy and capacity. They are important jointly as well as separately in that legitimacy speaks to the sanction now associated with such services and capacity speaks to the ability of systems to design and deliver services in an accountable fashion.

Standing in the way of further progress in home and community-based care development, however, are three sets of negative sectoral pressures: the still modest place of home and community-based care in the world of institutionally based long-term care; the lack of appreciation of the place and importance of long-term care in the constellation of social insurance activity; and, efforts to delegitimize social insurance protections of all sorts in broadscale debates about public policy and the role of government.

Further acceptance of home and community-based care in these ever-widening arenas is a daunting task. Indeed, in light of the 1994 elections and subsequent legislative proposals, it is difficult to generate great optimism about the home and community-based care policy future. Nonetheless, I suggest steps that will yield progress, at least if the larger environment does not become completely devolved and defunded. To the acute/long-term care divide, I suggest simply that client preferences and professional judgment should lead to more integrated and efficient care as institutional divisions are bridged. To the appropriate "nesting" of long-term care policy within social insurance protections, I suggest a two-part approach, centered on assessment of the particular risk characteristics associated with frailty and chronicity and, also, highlighting the successes in recent home and community-based care activity just reviewed. Well-designed home and community-based care programs—potentially spawned by the emerging combination of funding pressures and administrative flexibility—might show on however small a scale that governmentally sanctioned activities can be responsive, equitable, and cost-effective. They might counter the low esteem that public-sector activities generally enjoy today.

Finding an Expanded Place for HCBC in Long-Term Care

We have seen that considerable movement, certainly by historical comparison, has been made in the direction of home and community-based care within long-term care over the past several years. Between 1982 and 1990, Medicaid long-term care expenditures tilted, in proportional terms, clearly in the direction of noninstitutional care. This shift and the growing role of the 2176 waiver program and the personal care option under Medicaid is shown clearly in Nancy Miller's (1992) review of the waiver program experience (see Table 1). Medicaid expenditures for home and community-based care services increased over the eight-year period from $168 million to $3.9 billion. Coupled with the Older Americans Act, home and community-based care expenditures are estimated to be $765 million (U.S. GAO, 1991) and state-only expenditures will constitute $523 million. These figures demonstrate that meaningful amounts are now being placed into this service option.

Given the growing levels of severe frailty among an increasingly old population, nursing homes are under no threat of being supplanted, Medicaid cuts and block grants notwithstanding. In fact, the trend toward nursing homes caring for the increasingly frail will be exacerbated should major Medicaid long-term care cuts surface. That eventually will, in turn, make home and community settings ever more necessary for those whose incomes hover above the nursing home care threshold. Great demand will be present for home and community-based care services, and the battles over ever-tighter public funds will be intense. Yet, the appeal of services in

TABLE 1

Medicaid Long-Term Care Spending by Program, 1982

Skilled nursing facility	Intermediate care facility	Intermediate facility for mentally retarded	Home health	Total long-term care $$
39.1%	35.8%	23.9%	1.2%	$14,015

Medicaid Long-Term Care Spending by Program, 1990

Skilled nursing facility	Intermed. care facility	Intermed. care facility for mentally retarded	Home health	2176 waiver program	Personal care	Total long-term care $$
26.7%	34%	25.9%	2.8%	4.3%	6.3%	$29,423

the home and the development of intermediate service/dwelling options, such as assisted living and adult day care, make it hard to see a diminution of the home and community-based care "share" of long-term care service provision. Increased client cost-sharing and, ultimately, private insurance coverage will, however, represent a growing part of the funding picture.

Locating Long-Term Care Within Social Insurance

I have argued elsewhere (Hudson, 1993, 1995) the case for making chronic illness and disability coverage a matter deserving of more absolute and relative attention in our social insurance interventions. Based on the concept of risk or "social contingencies," the core argument is that not only do contemporary elders face chronic conditions in greater numbers than ever before but that the properties of functional incapacity, both their cost and their potential severity, make it an extremely appropriate candidate for expanded social insurance coverage. Using a typology of contingent events, I suggest that functional incapacity is today potentially more severe, more variable in its onset and duration, and more appropriately insured than are the other two great risks of old age–the need for income support and for acute care health coverage–which we currently cover relatively well. While I do not want to overstate this position–especially in light of current trends in private pension coverage–a strong case can be made to reweigh age-related social insurance coverage at least modestly in this direction.

Other analysts speak to the same point. Karen Holden and Timothy Smeeding (1990) note that economic well-being is about both being able to meet current consumption needs and having holdings that "can be drawn upon to cover the costs of uncertain contingencies." Nicholas Barr (1992) observes that modern welfare states have done remarkably well at "income smoothing," but less well at protecting established living standards against "unaccustomed drops," such as those very much associated with chronic incapacities. And, finally, it seems clear that Hugh Heclo's (1974) statement that social security is dependent on economic security, which is in turn dependent on income security, is not so nearly the case today as it was 20 years ago. In addition to normal consumption income, economic security is increasingly about adequate health and sickness coverage against potentially severe and unpredictable incapacities associated with very advanced age. "Social" security is about all that and, as well, a variety of additional housing and environmental supports. In short, the argument here suggests that we need to focus more attention on *what* protections we offer individuals and less on debates about *which individu-*

als we should bring under insurance coverage. Debates are now centered principally on presumptively unneeded protections offered the affluent.

These contentions underscore the changing face of risk in old age (and the ongoing underappreciation of the risk of disability among younger populations) and support a strong theoretical argument for greater long-term care protections. As events, frailty and disability have strong insurance imperatives; yet our social insurance protections barely scratch the surface of legitimate need while making rather ample provision for income support and acute health care needs.

One would like to think that improving the alignment between risk and coverage would be a winning social policy argument in the present budget-balancing environment. Unfortunately, placing a lessened emphasis on normal consumption income translates into an examination of the amount and distribution of Social Security benefits. The reluctance of politicians to engage in that examination is well-known. Indeed, one of the most dispiriting planks of House Speaker Newt Gingrich's Contract with America calls for raising the "retirement test" amounts under Social Security to $30,000 by the year 2002 (from today's $11,160) and rescinding the 1993 decision to tax 85% of Social Security benefits paid to very high-income recipients. Not only are these major expansions in benefits directed toward the wrong beneficiaries (those in the middle- and upper-income groups) but they are, as well, directed against the wrong risk–the need for consumption income rather than a lack of protection against selected discrete events.

Social Policy and the Public Sector

Hard as it would be to elevate long-term care concerns on the social insurance agenda, more difficult yet is it to come to grips with the public malaise centered on social intervention by government. As argued by John Myles (1984), we are living today in a political world where the pendulum is swinging in the direction of "economic liberalism" and away from "political democracy." After a half century's movement in the latter direction, the tide today is clearly in favor of allocating resources through markets rather than through governments. The macro-level evidence is, of course, pervasive as seen in the widespread ascendancy of conservative thinking and incumbency, the scaling back of welfare-state benefits, and policy initiatives more concerned with income generation than distribution.

Evidence at the micro level centers on questions of incentives, more particularly the "perverse" incentives of government programs that weaken notions of self-reliance and family responsibility. Especially interesting are arguments centered on so-called moral hazard, wherein, "the more complete the [insurance] cover . . . the less the individuals have to bear the consequences of their own actions and the less, therefore, the incentive to behave as they would if they had to bear the loss themselves" (Barr, 1992). Moral hazard is featured in critiques of virtually all coverage areas of contemporary social welfare: the poor and unemployed have insufficient incentives to work; clients and providers in health care have good reason to overutilize and to overserve; and those providing social services fare well while, wittingly or not, inducing their clients into "dependency relationships."

In a classic "good news/bad news" scenario, the old and, to a lesser extent, the impaired are now subject to moral hazard strictures. These were "deserving" recipient populations, once understood to be universally poor and sick, designations that vastly reduced concern about moral hazard. Those who are poor and sick deserve both income and care. However, now that members of these populations collectively are better off and/or better able to contribute to society, they, too, can fall victim to perverse incentives: cease working (retire too early), overconsume (fostering generational inequities), and overutilize benefits (lessen use of family or self-care).

These emergent macro- and micro-level concerns associated with the move toward Myles' economic liberalism have rather immediate effects on long-term care and home and community-based care in particular. At the macro level, budgets, allocations, and economic opportunity costs are the issues; at the micro level, loose eligibility criteria, substitution of formal/public for informal/private care, and fraud head the list of possible abuses.

As a result of these concerns, home and community-based care not only faces a new set of challenges to its expansion, it faces political pressures that were largely absent in the true expansionary phase of aging policy in the 1960s and 1970s. As variously argued by Theodore Marmor (1970) in the case of Medicare, Vincent Burke and Vee Burke in the case of Supplemental Security Income, and Robert Binstock (1972) in the case of the Older Americans Act, the deservingness of the old (or in SSI's case, the so-called "adult categories," including as well the blind and disabled) was based on common beliefs about their singular vulnerability. However, now that the old can "misbehave" in ways analogous to other recipients of public-sector benefits, home and community-based care expansion faces both micro- and macro-level barriers.

THE POLICY AND POLITICAL CONTRIBUTIONS OF HCBC

Home and community-based care has attained a new legitimacy and has demonstrated growing capacity as a system, and both of these developments should auger well for expanded utilization of such services. Recent political events, however, present a stunning challenge to expansions here as well as in numerous other areas of federal policy. The combination of program appeal and system capacity supports the contention that such services will grow. What remains unknown is what proportion of that growth will be as a result of the federal and state governments including it under their auspices and in their budgets. Clearly, Medicaid 2176 waivers have been popular, for reasons of both financing and flexibility. Should proposals (pending at this writing) to transform Medicaid into a block grant become law, complicated political questions will arise in the 50 states. As Justice (1995) observes, waiver programs are not entitlements, and there are clear Medicaid entitlements–largely for younger populations–under current law. How Medicaid home and community-based care programs should fare and will fare are extremely important questions in this truly "dedistributive" (Light, 1985) environment.

Rather than speculate further along these lines, it simply remains to be restated that there are today intrinsic reasons to call for and defend home and community-based care expansion. Especially in such politically constrained times, it is important to be able to make such a statement with so little equivocation.

REFERENCES

Alter, C.F. (1988). The changing structure of elderly service delivery systems. *The Gerontologist*, *28*, 91-98.

Barr, N. (1992). Economic theory and the welfare state. *Journal of Economic Literature*, *30*, 741-803.

Benjamin, A.E. (1993). An historical perspective on home care policy. *Milbank Quarterly*, *71*, 129-166.

Binstock, R.H. (1972). Interest group liberalism and the politics of aging. *The Gerontologist*, *12*, 265-280.

Burke, V., & Burke, V. (1974). *Nixon's good deed*. New York: Columbia University Press.

Derthick, M. (1990). *Agency under stress: The Social Security Administration in American government*. Washington, DC: Brookings Institution.

Derthick, M. (1975). *Uncontrollable spending for social services grants*. Washington, DC: Brookings Institution.

Fortinksy, R.H. (1991). Coordinated, comprehensive, coordinated community care and the Older Americans Act. *Generations*, *15* (3), 39-42.

Haber, C. (1993, Summer/Fall). "And the fear of the poor house": Perceptions of old age impoverishment in early twentieth-century America. *Generations*, *17*, 46-50.

Heclo, H. (1974). *Modern social politics in Britain and Sweden*. New Haven, CT: Yale University Press.

Holden, K.C., & Smeeding, T.M. (1990). The poor, the rich, and the insecure elderly caught in between. *Milbank Quarterly, 68*, 191-220.

Hudson, R.B. (1983). *Strategies for capacity-building in the aging network*. Report submitted to the U.S. Administration on Aging pursuant to Award 90AM0029/01.

Hudson, R.B. (1993). Social contingencies, the aged, and public policy. *Milbank Quarterly, 71*, 253-277.

Hudson, R.B. (1995). The evolution of the welfare state: Shifting rights and responsibilities for the old. *International Social Security Review, 48* (1), 3-17.

Justice, D. (1988). *State long-term care reform: Development of community care systems in six states*. Washington, DC: National Governors Association.

Justice, D. (1995). *Changes in Medicaid: Implications for state units on aging*. Presentation to the annual meeting of the National Association of State Units on Aging, Washington, DC, June 14.

Kane, R.A., Penrod, J.D., Davidson, G., Moscovice, I., & Rich, E. (1991). What cost case management in long-term care? *Social Service Review, 65*, 281-303.

Kane, R.A., Urv-Wong, K., & King. C. (Eds.). (1990). *Case management: What is it anyway*? Minneapolis: University of Minnesota Long-Term Care DECISIONS Resource Center.

Kavesh, W.N. (1986). Home care: Process, outcome, cost. *Annual Review of Gerontology and Geriatrics* (Vol. 6). New York: Springer.

Leutz, W., Abrahams, R., & Capitman, J. (1993). The administration of eligibility for community long-term care. *The Gerontologist, 33*, 92-104.

Light, P. (1985). *Artful work*. New York: Random House.

Lubove, R. (1968). *The struggle for Social Security*. Cambridge, MA.: Harvard University Press.

Marmor, T.R. (1970). *The politics of Medicare*. Chicago: Aldine.

Miller, N.A. (1992). Medicaid 2176 home and community-based care waivers. *Health Affairs, 11* (4), 162-171.

Mundlinger, M.O. (1983). *Home care controversies*. Rockville, MD: Aspen Systems.

Myles, J. (1984). *Old age in the welfare state*. Boston: Little Brown.

O'Shaughnessy, C. (1991). *Targeting services to older persons under Title III of the Older Americans Act*. Washington, DC: Congressional Research Service.

Quirk, D. (1991). The aging network: An agenda for the nineties and beyond. *Generations, 15* (3), 23-26.

Smith, S. R., & Lipsky, M. (1992). *Non-profits for hire*. Cambridge, MA: Harvard University Press.

Stone, R., & Murtaugh, C.M. (1990). The elderly population with chronic functional disability: Implications for home care eligibility. *The Gerontologist, 30*, 491-496.

Sundquist, J. (1968). *Politics and policy: The Eisenhower, Kennedy, and Johnson years*. Washington, DC: Brookings Institution.

Torres-Gil, F., & Pynoos, J. (1986). Long-term care policy and interest group struggles. *The Gerontologist*, *26*, 488-495.

U.S. General Accounting Office. (1991). *Administration on Aging: More federal action needed to promote service coordination for the elderly*. Washington, DC: Author.

U.S. General Accounting Office. (1994). *Long-term care: Status of quality assurance and measurement in home and community-based services*. Washington, DC: Author.

Vladeck, B. (1980). *Unloving care*. New York: Basic Books.

Informal Care vs. Formal Services: Changes in Patterns of Care Over Time

Sharon Tennstedt, PhD
Brooke Harrow, PhD
Sybil Crawford, PhD
New England Research Institutes
Watertown, Massachusetts

SUMMARY. Longitudinal data from a representative sample of community-residing older persons were used to document changes in patterns and costs of care, both informal and formal. It was found that use of formal services was usually in conjunction with, and secondary to, informal care. Limited availability of informal care as well as increased disability raised the odds of using services. Substitution of formal services for informal care was limited and usually temporary. Total costs of community care, including living expenses, were generally less than the cost of nursing home care. *[Article copies available from The Haworth Document Delivery Service: 1-800-342-9678.]*

Sharon Tennstedt is a Senior Research Scientist and Director of the Institute for Studies on Aging at the New England Research Institutes (NERI). Her major research interests include caregiving systems for community-residing disabled elders, doctor-patient relationships, and community intervention trials to enhance independent functioning. Brooke Harrow is a Senior Research Scientist and Health Economist at NERI. Her work focuses on cost-benefit and cost-effectiveness analyses. Sybil Crawford, also a Senior Research Scientist and a Statistician at NERI, directs longitudinal analyses for several NERI studies and is recognized for her work in handling missing data and nonrandom attrition.

This work was supported by National Institute on Aging Grant No. AG07182.

The authors may be contacted care of the New England Research Institutes, 9 Galen Street, Watertown, MA 02172.

[Haworth co-indexing entry note]: "Informal Care vs. Formal Services: Changes in Patterns of Care Over Time." Tennstedt, Sharon, Brooke Harrow, and Sybil Crawford. Co-published simultaneously in *Journal of Aging & Social Policy* (The Haworth Press, Inc.) Vol. 7, No. 3/4, 1996, pp. 71-91; and: *From Nursing Homes to Home Care* (ed: Marie E. Cowart and Jill Quadagno) The Haworth Press, Inc., 1996, pp. 71-91. Single or multiple copies of this article are available from The Haworth Document Delivery Service [1-800-342-9678, 9:00 a.m. - 5:00 p.m. (EST)].

According to the National Academy of Aging (1994, p. 4), "[h]ealth care costs of older people have been depicted as a great fiscal 'black hole', posing an unsustainable burden for the economy." This statement might also be true for costs of long-term care–particularly community-based services. This fiscal black hole is even more of an unknown because of both the current sources and delivery of community care. It is widely acknowledged that at least 80% of long-term care assistance for the estimated 5.5 million functionally dependent older persons in this country (Leon & Lair, 1990) is provided informally at no public cost (Spillman & Kemper, 1992). Relatively few dependent elders rely exclusively on formal services to meet their needs (Liu, Manton, & Liu, 1985). Rather, it is much more common for disabled elders to receive *both* informal care and formal services (Soldo, Wolf, & Agree, 1989; Tennstedt, Sullivan, McKinlay, & D'Agostino, 1990), especially if needs for care are extensive (Kemper, 1992; Macken, 1986; Tennstedt et al., 1990) or if elders have a higher income level (Liu et al., 1985).

The role of informal helpers is clearly critical to maintaining a functionally dependent elder in the community. At the present time, formal services play a much more limited and supplementary role than do informal services. Even when an older person receives both kinds of care, informal care predominates (Noelker & Wallace, 1985; Tennstedt et al., 1990). The growing recognition of the major role of these uncompensated helpers fuels the continued concern with the great fiscal "black hole" of long-term care.

The concern emanates from suggestions regarding who will need and use formal–specifically, publicly funded–long-term care services. A fairly large body of literature exists regarding factors associated with formal service use, but the vast majority of information comes from cross-sectional studies and studies of nonrepresentative samples of elders. Data from these studies indicate that utilization is strongly associated with need but mediated by the availability of informal care (Evashwick, Rowe, Diehr, & Branch, 1984; McAuley & Arling, 1984; Soldo et al., 1990; Wan & Arling, 1983). However, what these cross-sectional studies have not been able to address adequately is what happens with utilization when there are changes in the availability or provision of informal care. The future availability and resilience of informal care has been called into question repeatedly in the last decade (Doty, 1986; Hanley, Weiner, & Harris, 1991; Stone & Kemper, 1989; U. S. General Accounting Office, 1988), usually on the basis of several social trends undergoing change. Related to this is the question of what might happen with utilization–and the provision of informal care–given the widespread availability of community long-term care services. That is, if formal services were more readily available, would families withdraw their unpaid help and use services to meet the care needs of the elder?

The answers to these questions might serve to diminish fears concerning the depth and likelihood of the dreaded fiscal black hole of community long-term care. Data reported here attempt to supply some answers; they come from a longitudinal study of a representative sample of disabled older persons and their informal caregivers designed to investigate changes in the caregiving pattern over a seven-year period (1984-1991). The study was conducted in Massachusetts, a state that provides a comprehensive array of case-managed community services at no cost to low-income elders and on a sliding-fee basis to others. Therefore, locating the study in Massachusetts permitted an investigation of changes in informal care in the context of publicly funded services. This is an important point since data from the National Long-Term Care Demonstration Program have shown that the probability of individuals using services and, if used, the number of hours of service used are greater where there is a state home-care program (Kemper, 1992). In addition, the availability of detailed data regarding both the amount and type of formal services and informal care permits an examination of the changes in each source of care vis-à-vis the other over time, as well as an estimation of the costs of each source and type of care.

More specifically, the objectives of the analyses reported in this article were to document the changes in patterns of care over time and the factors–both physical and social–that are associated with these changes. Those investigated in the study included:

- A change from predominantly informal care to predominantly formal care, and specifically the substitution of formal services for informal care;
- The initiation of formal services for someone receiving informal care;
- The initiation of formal services where there was no informal care; and
- Termination of community care because the person was admitted to a nursing home.

In addition, because of the specific interest in the costs of potential increases in formal service use, cost estimates were developed to compare the following:

- Changes in the costs of community care for elders where formal services were substituted and where they were not; and

- Costs of community care for elders in the case of total substitution of formal services versus costs of institutional care.

METHODS

Sample

The Massachusetts Elder Health Project is a longitudinal study of a representative sample of older people which investigated their needs for assistance with daily living activities (ADLs) and sources (both formal and informal) and patterns of the help received. Data used in this article were collected at four points in time (1984-85, 1988-89, 1990-91, 1991) from both functionally disabled elders and their primary informal caregivers. A geographically stratified random sample of 5,855 older adults 70 years old and older was drawn in two stages, using towns and cities of eastern Massachusetts as the primary sampling unit (PSU) and then randomly selecting individuals within these PSUs. The samples used in these analyses consisted of elders who were disabled and residing in the community for at least two sequential points of contact. Characteristics of the samples of elders at each of the three transitions are summarized in Table 1; the size and characteristics of the transition samples vary because each sample consists of surviving respondents who were disabled at both waves, comprising each transition period. Further description of the sampling strategy, response rates, and field methods can be found in Tennstedt, Crawford, and McKinlay (1993).

Measures

Baseline data were collected in 1984-1985 on the initial sample of 4,185 eligible individuals (response rate = 87.7%). Each of the three follow-up interviews were conducted at 15-month intervals starting in 1988. Because of the longitudinal nature of the data, two forms of notations are used to describe the points of contact and transition periods between contact. The specific points of contact are referred to as baseline, FU1, FU2, and FU3. Regarding any transition between points of contact, T_i refers to the earlier point of contact and $T_i + 1$ to the subsequent point of contact.

Outcome measures. Data used to detect patterns of care consisted of the types and amounts (average hours per week in the month prior to interview) of informal care provided by the primary caregiver and up to three

TABLE 1. Sample Characteristics at Each Transition
Percentage of Disabled Elders at Both Contacts

	BL and FU1 (N = 236)	FU1 and FU2 (N = 300)	FU2 and FU3 (N = 232)
T_i disability level:			
Minimal	30.1	32.3	12.5
Moderate	8.1	20.3	26.3
Severe	33.9	26.6	29.7
Extreme	19.9	13	16.8
Very extreme	8.1	8	14.7
Cognitive Impairment at T_i	7.6	20.5	21.5
Gender: Male	14	16.6	19.7
Annual Income			
< $5000	28.8	12.6	13.3
$5000-$10,000	63.1	75.5	60.1
> $10,000	8.1	11.9	26.6
Coresidence with PCG[a] at T_i	42.4	44.2	47.8
Relationship to T_i PCG[a]:			
Spouse	22.9	17.3	20.3
Offspring	42.4	47	49.1
Other relative	17.8	21	19
Nonrelative	11.9	4.7	3.4
No T_i PCG	5.1	10	8.2
Change in disability:			
Less	31.8	17.7	14.2
Same	35.6	36.7	41.8
More	32.6	45.7	844
Change in Cognitive Impairment			
No > Yes	17.4	11.6	13.3
Yes > No	2.1	6.3	7.7
No Change	80.5	82.1	79.0

[a]PCG = Primary caregiver

TABLE 1 (continued)

	BL and FU1 (N = 236)	FU1 and FU2 (N = 300)	FU2 and FU3 (N = 232)
Number of CGs at T_i			
0	5.1	10.0	8.2
1	16.9	37.5	30.2
≥2	78.0	52.5	61.6
Change in # of CGs at $T_i + 1$			
Fewer	48.7	22.7	20.3
Same	39.8	43.7	38.5
More	11.4	33.7	41.1
Change in PCG:			
No PCG > No PCG	3.0	5.6	4.7
Different PCG	19.9	20.9	15.0
No PCG > PCG	2.1	4.3	3.4
PCG > No PCG	11.4	2.6	2.6
Same PCG	63.6	66.5	74.2
Change in Residence:			
Alone > Alone	50.8	46.4	49.4
Alone > with PCG	6.8	8.9	2.6
With PCG > Alone	8.9	5.3	5.2
With PCG > with PCG	33.5	39.4	42.9

Note: Percentages may not add to 100% due to rounding.

secondary caregivers as well as the types and amounts (average hours per week in the month prior to interview) of formal services utilized. Six common types of assistance were investigated, matching informal care with a formal service as indicated in Table 2. Formal services could be arranged from public or private agencies or on a private-hire basis.

These hours of informal care and formal services were used to define *primary source of care* as follows:

- Informal only: No formal services
- Formal services only: No informal care

- Mixed care: Both informal care and formal services
  - Predominantly informal: Hours of informal care > hours of formal services
  - Predominantly formal: Hours of formal services > hours of informal care.

The *substitution of formal services for informal care* from any one period to the next (i.e., T_i to $T_i + 1$) was defined as occurring when the following two conditions were satisfied:

- Hours of formal service at $T_i + 1 >$ hours of formal service at T_i
- Hours of informal care at $T_i + 1 <$ hours of informal care at T_i

That is, from one period to the next, the amount of formal assistance increased while the amount of informal care decreased. In order to detect true substitution, the possibility that caregivers redistributed their time to other areas of ADL assistance (*specialization of informal care*) was also investigated, with the omission of these cases from the analysis (see Tennstedt et al., 1993 for further detail).

Cost of informal caregiving. The cost of informal caregiving hours was calculated by imputing the market value of the services provided. This approach captures the economic costs of informal caregiving time by using a wage rate for paid employees providing similar services (Hu, Huang, &

TABLE 2. Types of Informal Care and Formal Services

Informal Care	Formal Services
Personal care	Home health aide or nurse
Housekeeping	Homemaker or chore
Meals	Home-delivered or congregate meals
Transportation	Transportation service, taxi, ambulance
Managing finances	Financial management, Accountant, lawyer
Arranging services	Case management

Cartwright, 1986; Max, Webber, & Fox, 1995; Rice et al., 1993). The Bureau of Labor Statistics (U.S. Department of Labor, 1993) median wage rate for comparable occupations was used for each of the six areas of care studied. The median wage rate for a nurse's aide was used for personal care and transportation hours. "Private household cleaners and servants" was the occupational group selected for housekeeping and meals. The median wage for bookkeepers and the median wage for social workers were selected for hours of financial assistance and arranging services, respectively. These figures were inflated to account for fringe benefits, adjusted to reflect Massachusetts area wages and converted to 1991 dollars using the Consumer Price Index. The adjusted hourly wage rates used in the analysis can be found in Harrow, Tennstedt and McKinlay (1995).

Cost of formal services. For formal services, we used the average charge per hour for each type of formal service, when possible. Available rates for 1994 were deflated to 1991 dollars and used for all three time periods. The hourly rate for "homemaker service" in Massachusetts (Executive Office of Elder Affairs, personal communication, 1994) was used for housekeeping and meals. The hourly rate for a "home health aide worker" (Massachusetts Rate Setting Commission, personal communication, 1994) was used for personal care and transportation. For case management services and financial services, the same adjusted wage rates were used as for the informal hours.

Predictor variables. Potential predictors of patterns or changes in source of care included both elder and caregiver factors. These variables were selected primarily because of previously reported associations with the provision of informal care or utilization of formal services (c.f. Horowitz, 1985; Tennstedt et al., 1990). Elder factors included (a) two measures of the elder's disability status, the *level of disability* at T_i (a 5-point scale ranging from minimal to very extreme) and *change in the level of disability* at $T_i + 1$ (less disabled, no change, more disabled); (b) *cognitive impairment* at T_i (coded "yes" if either the elder reported frequent confusion or if a proxy interview was required because of cognitive impairment; coded "no" otherwise), and *change in cognitive impairment status* at $T_i + 1$; (c) *elder gender*; (d) *living arrangement* including any change from one period to the next (lives alone, moves from living with a caregiver to living alone, moves from living alone to living with a caregiver); and (e) *elder annual income* at T_i. Caregiver factors included an interaction term of *caregiver relationship* at T_i and his or her *coresidence status* with the elder (coresiding offspring, noncoresiding offspring, coresiding other relative, noncoresiding other relative, noncoresiding nonrelative; spouses were the referent group). Other caregiver factors included a *change in primary caregiver* from T_i to $T_i + 1$ (lose caregiver, different caregiver) and any *change in the number of caregivers* from T_i to $T_i + 1$ (fewer, no change, more).

Because primary caregivers providing many hours of informal care might feel burdened and are therefore likely to substitute formal services for some of their care, the *log informal hours at* T_i for each of the six types of care, as well as *total amount of care*, were included as potential predictors in the models investigating service substitution. The log of hours was used instead of simply hours of care in order to reduce the influence of outlying values, as well as to satisfy the requirement of linearity in the statistical models. Finally, because of the difference in length of time between contacts (i.e., four years between baseline and follow-up compared with approximately 15 months between subsequent follow-up contacts), we also included indicators (1 = yes, 0 = no) for each transition (baseline to FU1, FU1 to FU2, and FU2 to FU3). This provided a better fit to the data than did including the elapsed time between T_i and $T_i + 1$.

ANALYSIS

To address the study objectives, the analyses consisted of comparison rates of change in various patterns of care across the three transition periods, that is, BL to FU1, FU1 to FU2, and FU2 to FU3.

Then, to identify predictors of various changes in patterns of care, a logistic regression model was developed for each specific type of change. The sample for each model consisted of elders who were functionally disabled at the start of the study or, FU1 or FU2, and who remained disabled and still residing in the community at the following interview. Cases in which the loss of the primary caregiver was experienced (n = 19) were dropped from these models because any elder who lost his or her caregiver switched to predominantly formal services or no care. If these cases had been included in the models, with loss of caregiver as a predictor, there would have been numerical problems in estimation of the model, since the probability of this change = 1 in all cases. These 19 cases, however, were included in the calculation of rates.

Next, elder and caregiver characteristics associated with substitution were identified by estimating a multiple logistic regression model for the probability of substitution, taking each area of need separately. The sample for each model consisted of elders who received the relevant type of informal care at baseline, FU1 or FU2, and who remained disabled and residing in the community at the subsequent interview.

Because of the large number of potential explanatory variables, we employed stepwise modeling to identify a parsimonious model; such a procedure eliminates irrelevant or redundant predictor variables in stages, thereby allowing better estimation of the effects of the remaining covariates (Hosmer & Lemeshow, 1989). The fit of the estimated model to the study data was assessed using the Hosmer-Lemeshow goodness-of-fit chi-square statistic (Hosmer, Taber, & Lemeshow, 1989).[1] Some elders contributed more than one observation to these analyses because the individuals were interviewed up to four times. To account for the dependence between repeated measurements on the same subject, the standard errors of the parameter estimates were adjusted, using a procedure that involved the correlation of multiple residuals from the same subject similar to calculation of design effects in cluster sampling (see Liang & Zeger, 1986; Lipsitz & Harrington, 1990). Exploratory analyses indicated that the relationship between substitution status and predictors was stable over time, so that combining the three datasets (baseline to FU1, FU1 to FU2, FU2 to FU3) into a single model was appropriate.

Finally, to investigate costs associated with the formal services for informal care substitution, the average hours of care and cost of care were compared between elders who had experienced service substitution and those who had not. Cost of care was calculated by applying the wage rates previously stated to the hours of care. Informal, formal, and total hours of care were computed separately for comparison across the two groups.

The total cost for complete service substitution was simulated. The simulation analysis assumed that the total hours of care remained constant from T_i to $T_i + 1$. In $T_i + 1$, all these hours were assumed to be for formal services, and the formal service hourly rates were used to calculate the total cost. The simulated costs were then compared to the costs of institutionalization.

RESULTS

Rates of Change in Source of Care

Looking first at the changes in patterns of care, results are displayed in Table 3. Again, because it is well established that informal care predominates for the vast majority of elders, the study examined changes in the use of formal services vis-à-vis informal care. These data indicate that a relatively small proportion (12%-17%) of elders turned from reliance on informal care to reliance on formal services for needed help and that the likelihood of this pattern of change decreased over time. In contrast, more elders (35%-40%) were likely to change from relying on formal services to relying on informal care.

At each transition period, just over one third (33%-39%) of elders receiving informal care also began using formal services, and the proportion of elders who started formal service use increased over time (Table 3). The number of elders who began service use *without* receiving any informal care as well, however, was quite low, particularly at later waves of the study when these elders were more disabled. Therefore, while we see an increased tendency on the part of older people to use formal services, in almost all cases it is in conjunction with informal care. That is, formal services complement informal care.

Looking specifically at whether formal services substituted for, or replaced, informal care, data in Table 3 show that, after omitting elders who experienced specialization of informal care (having their caregivers redistribute their time to other ADL assistance), the rates of overall service substitution ranged from 14% to 20%. Findings from previous analyses (Tennstedt et al., 1993) suggest that when service substitution occurred, it did so in all areas of informal care. That is, very little care specialization by informal caregivers occurred. Rates of service substitution from baseline to FU1 tended to be somewhat higher than at subsequent periods. This

TABLE 3. Rates of Change in Source of Care

	Transition Period		
	BL FU1 % (n)	FU1 FU2 % (n)	FU2 FU3 % (n)
Change in Care Mix			
Mostly informal to mostly formal	17.2 (29)	12.5 (29)	11.7 (21)
Mostly formal to mostly informal	34.8 (23)	33.3 (22)	44.0 (22)
Initiation of Formal Services			
With informal care	33.3 (23)	35.8 (43)	38.6 (32)
Without informal care	12.1 (27)	3.3 (9)	3.3 (7)
Service Substitution[a]	19.7 (30)	13.8 (27)	14.9 (23)

[a]Elders with any specialization of care are omitted.

higher rate of service substitution is most likely related to the longer time period between baseline and FU1. The rates of service substitution for the next two transition periods are fairly consistent and more likely provide a closer estimate of how much substitution of formal services for informal care occurs annually.

Predictors of Changes in Care Pattern

Change from predominantly informal care to reliance on formal services (Table 4) was predicted by an increase in disability, living alone, move from coresidence with a caregiver to living alone, and having a coresiding caregiver who was not a close relative. The living arrangement of the elder is particularly important here, with those living alone being four to eight times more likely to rely on formal services than those living with others.

There were actually two potential scenarios for these elders in terms of the amount of their informal care: (1) the amount of informal care could have also increased or remained the same, or (2) the amount of informal care could have decreased, representing a substitution of formal services. Reliance on formal services with an increase or no change in informal care was predicted only in the instance of people living alone. The results of the logistic regression model (Table 4) indicate that the most consistent predictor of service substitution was the loss of the primary caregiver. Depending on the type of care, elders who lost a primary caregiver were between nine and 35 times as likely to substitute formal services for informal assistance. To a lesser degree, elders with a different primary caregiver at T_i also had higher rates of substitution. Other important predictors of service substitution included living alone at $T_i + 1$, particularly a change of coresidence at T_i to living alone at $T_i + 1$. Elders who lived alone and had an other-relative primary caregiver at T_i also had a higher rate of service substitution in the area of arranging services. While there were some differences in predictors of service substitution across various types of care (Tennstedt et al., 1993), overall factors associated with the availability of a caregiver (i.e., loss of a caregiver and living alone) increased the odds of substituting formal services for informal care to a much greater extent than did a greater need for care.

A similar pattern emerges in terms of factors that predict initiation of formal service use. Predictors of starting the use of formal services are displayed in Table 4, and include greater disability, living alone, and having a change in primary caregiver. However, having an adult-child caregiver, even though that person may not be coresident, decreases the chance of an older person's starting service use. Almost all cases in which

TABLE 4. Significant Predictors of Three Types of Changes in Pattern of Informal Care and Formal Services: Odds Ratios (95% C. I.)

	Changes in Pattern of Care		
Predictor	Predominantly Informal to Predominantly Formal	Substitution of Formal Services[b]	Initiation of Formal Services
Disability Level Increase	1.84 (1.04, 3.25)	1.74 (1.02, 2.96)	2.04 (1.22, 3.41)
Relationship to T_i PCG			
Nonresident offspring			0.34 (0.14, 0.81)
Coresident other relative	2.87 (1.30, 8.03)		
Living Situation			
Living alone > Living alone	7.67 (3.76, 15.67)	3.51 (1.62, 7.59)	3.29 (1.38, 7.85)
Co-reside > Live alone	3.87 (1.26, 11.86)	4.39 (1.79, 10.79)	
Change in PCG			
Different PCG		2.30 (1.22, 4.36)	2.62 (1.12, 6.14)
Loss of PCG		10.18 (4.45, 23.29)	
T_i Informal Hours[a]			
Log total hours		3.51 (2.04, 6.01)	

[a]Evaluated at increase from 25th percentile to 75th percentile
[b]Elders with specialization of care were omitted from this model

formal services were initiated in the absence of informal care occurred when the elder reported they had lost a caregiver and had no replacement for that person.

Costs of Care

Table 5 presents the average informal, formal, and total hours of care and costs of care separately for those elders who experienced no substitution of formal services for informal care and those who did have service substitution. For those elders with *no service substitution*, average use of both informal and formal services increased slightly during the transition period from FU1 to FU2. Informal care hours for the six service areas combined increased from an average of 17.2 to 18.2 hours per week. The total formal service hours increased about 1 hour per week, from 3 to 4 hours. This change was fairly consistent across types of care, with the exception of housekeeping and meals. For these two areas, total care hours declined between FU1 and FU2.

When *substitution of formal services* for informal services occurred, total hours of care decreased by one third from FU1 to FU2. Average informal care hours dropped from 17 to a little over 6 hours per week. Formal services did not fill this gap; they increased only from 4 to 8 hours

TABLE 5. Total Hours and Cost Per Week of Care, by Source of Care and Service Substitution Status, for Two Transition Periods

Status		FU1 to FU2					
		Informal		Formal		Total	
		Hours	Cost	Hours	Cost	Hours	Cost
No Service Substitution	FU1	17.21	$129.93	3.01	$38.52	20.22	$168.45
	FU2	18.18	$136.70	4.07	$51.09	22.25	$187.79
Service Substitution	FU1	16.97	$130.58	4.12	$54.18	21.09	$184.76
	FU2	6.39	$63.28	8.12	$81.97	14.51	$145.25
		FU2 to FU3					
No Service Substitution	FU2	17.34	$133.78	3.96	$44.50	21.29	$178.28
	FU3	20.79	$162.24	3.97	$50.57	24.76	$212.81
Service Substitution	FU2	21.28	$161.98	4.81	$59.08	26.10	$221.06
	FU3	7.66	$66.47	9.10	$142.99	16.76	$209.46

per week. However, total hours of care did not decline for each type of care. The data indicate that personal care hours remained constant, and total hours spent arranging services actually doubled. This increase in hours arranging services was almost entirely due to an increase in informal care, perhaps accounted for by the caregiver time necessary to coordinate the increase in formal services.

Results for the transition from FU2 to FU3 were similar as also shown in Table 5. During this transition period, total caregiving hours for those elders with no substitution also increased. This was entirely due to increased informal care. For those elders who had service substitution, total caregiving hours again decreased one third, from an average 26 hours a week to under 17 hours. Results were fairly consistent by type of care, with the exception of personal care and housekeeping, where the total hours received increased during this transition.

As expected from the data presented on hours, average costs for those elders who experienced service substitution declined over both transition periods, while the average total costs of caregiving for those elders with no service substitution increased. These data suggest that the total costs of care were less with substitution of formal services for informal care than with no substitution if the costs of informal care are included in the total. Primarily, this was because fewer total hours of care were provided following service substitution. As expected, the costs of formal services alone were higher in those cases with service substitution than those without substitution.

The study also was planned to try to determine whether or not the use of formal services would be cost-effective relative to institutionalization, even if no informal care is provided and there is a complete substitution of formal service hours for all informal care hours. Table 6 presents the results of a simulation of the scenario of total substitution of formal services for informal care for both transition periods (FU1 to FU2 and FU2 to FU3, respectively). The hours in the second column represent the total hours of care in T_i, for each type of service and in total, which in this simulation remain constant during the transition to $T_i + 1$. Therefore, the hours for T_i represent the actual hours (as reported by the caregiver) of both informal and formal care. For $T_i + 1$, the simulated hours are *all* formal service hours (i.e., replacing all hours of informal care with an equal number of hours of formal service). The third column of the table has the average weekly cost for T_i and the simulated average weekly cost for $T_i + 1$. The difference in cost between the two time periods in the simulation depends upon the difference in the hourly rates that were imputed for the informal care and formal service hours.

TABLE 6. Comparison of Costs for Community Services versus Nursing Home Care, Simulated for Cases of Total Substitution of Formal Services for Informal Care

Wave	Hours	Weekly Cost	Annual Cost	Annual Nursing Home Cost
FU1	21.09	$184.76	$9,608	$34,087
FU2		$286.18[a]	$14,877[a]	$35,522
FU2	26.10	$221.06	$11,495	$35,522
FU3		$327.66[a]	$17,038[a]	$35,522

[a]Simulated costs

The fourth column presents the "average annual costs," calculated by multiplying the average weekly cost by 52. For FU2 and FU3, the simulated total annual costs for caregiving with total substitution of informal caregiving for formal services were $14,877 and $17,038 respectively. The average cost per day in a nursing home in Massachusetts was $93.39 in 1990 (AARP, 1993), or $35,522 annually (in 1991 dollars). While the costs of community services were about 50% greater than those for the previous period, they were less than half of the cost of institutionalization.

Obviously, included in the total cost of nursing home care is food and shelter, which was not included in the total cost of community formal services. However, if these costs are added to the total annual costs in the simulation, the community-care setting was still far less expensive. For example, the average annual out-of-pocket expenditures for food and shelter for a single person in 1990, as taken from the Consumer Expenditure Survey (U.S. Department of Commerce, 1992) was $7,209, after adjusting for the Massachusetts area expenditures and inflating up to 1991 dollars. In fact, annual expenditures on food and shelter plus any other caregiving activities not already captured, would have to amount to $21,000 in order for the total costs in the community to equal the expense of a nursing home.

DISCUSSION

Several major points about the patterns of care for disabled elders over time could be drawn from these findings:

- Informal care remained the predominant source of help over time for most disabled elders.

- Formal services were most often used in conjunction with informal care.
- The use of formal services–whether initiated or increased–was associated with increased disability. However, social factors related to the availability of informal care increased the odds of using formal services more than disability did.
- There was no evidence of a major or persistent trend of replacement of informal care by formal services.
- For the most part, service substitution was temporary and related to the lack of an available caregiver at a point in time.
- Service substitution resulted in substantially higher formal service costs. However, even when assuming total substitution of formal services for informal care, annual costs of community care were substantially less than for nursing home care.

The findings regarding costs of care–and particularly costs of formal services–in the cases of formal service substitution were particularly interesting. These data indicate that when costs of informal or "unpaid" caregiving time were considered along with formal service costs, substitution of formal services for informal caregiving actually decreased the total costs of community-based care, although the total costs of formal services obviously increased. Specifically, when the number of informal hours declined and the formal service hours increased, less care was provided in total, because not every informal care hour was replaced by formal services.

There are several possible reasons for this decline in total care:

Access to formal services might have been limited. This study was conducted in a state with a well-established, publicly funded home care program. This remains true; in 1992, Massachusetts was ranked seventh with respect to home and community-based services expenditures per capita (Administration on Aging, 1994). It is unlikely that limitations related to access to services would be an explanation for the reduction in total hours of care. Furthermore, there was no evidence that elders with overall service substitution had greater unmet need than those elders with no substitution.

Those elders with service substitution were less frail and needed fewer total hours of care. This also did not appear to be true. In fact, the data indicated that an increase in disability was linked to overall service substitution (Tennstedt et al., 1993).

Formal services might be more efficient than informal services. This may be true. That is, hours of informal care and hours of formal service are not time-equivalent. The use of formal services such as housekeeping might require fewer number of hours due to the relative efficiency of the professional performing the service as compared to the informal caregiver. Or perhaps the time reported by informal caregivers for a task such as housekeeping includes time spent socializing with the care recipient as well.

Informal caregiving might be preferred to formal services. In this study, elders incurred either no or low out-of-pocket expenses for formal services and presumably no out-of-pocket expenses for informal services. When formal services are substituted for informal services, fewer hours may be consumed because of the preferences of the elder. For example, the elder might prefer fewer hours of help with housekeeping from an agency than from a family member because the help is provided by a stranger.

If elders do prefer informal caregiving services, then why does service substitution occur at all? It is important to restate that this study was conducted in a state with a well-established, publicly funded home care program, which would have made substitution of formal services for informal care easier. However, the fact that service substitution was temporary and related to the availability of the primary caregiver (Tennstedt et al., 1993) suggests that public funding for home care does not result in widespread and undesired (i.e., costly) service substitution. Publicly funded services appear to be doing what they are intended to do: supporting and sustaining the informal caregiving arrangement or providing care during the disruption (usually temporary) of the regular arrangement in order to keep the elder in the community. It cannot be denied that this substitution of formal services for previously provided informal care incurs costs that would not have been required had the informal care not been interrupted. However, the probable benefits of these services to both the care recipient, who desires to remain living at home, and to society, in containing the number of institutionalizations, appear to justify the costs.

It must be emphasized that these data reflect what is happening currently, not what is projected for the future. It is the changing social trends of increased female participation in the work force, decreasing fertility rates, increasing geographic mobility, and rising rates of marital disruption that result in the questions about the continued future availability of informal care. However, existing empirical evidence from investigations of caregiving does not unequivocally support the projected negative impact of these trends on a family's willingness to provide continued care (Tennstedt et al., 1993). Over 25 years, studies have consistently documented that the primary motivation for providing care is a sense of filial or familial responsibility (Horowitz, 1985; McKinlay & Tennstedt, 1986; Shanas et al., 1968; Sussman, 1979). It seems that the social trends in question would have to result in an erosion of this obligation before any widespread abandonment of the caregiving role would be seen. Families give care and likely will continue to give care. Formal services are being used and will continue to be used. Clearly, services will more likely be used and to a greater extent by elders with limited or no informal care resources. Based on results from this study, the current targeting in many states of home and community-based services to this population is highly appropriate and effective.

Not considered here, however, is the care recipient's perspective and preferences. That is, who makes the decision to use formal services–the care recipient or the caregiver? If it is the caregiver, data reported above suggest that home and community-based service use in the future will be minimal or used only when necessary. However, if the care recipient makes the decision, a different scenario might develop. Any new initiative expanding public long-term financing would increase eligibility for public benefits that disabled elders might choose to access rather than to ask offspring or other family members for assistance. Baseline data from this study revealed that 37% of disabled elders thought that they had the primary responsibility for their own care, with another 42% seeing the government as being responsible (McKinlay & Tennstedt, 1986). The latter group saw using formal services as a way to maintain independence.

Assuming that future cohorts of older persons will be better educated and have greater financial resources than current cohorts, this sense of responsibility for one's self might be even more prevalent. This suggests that use of formal services might increase for reasons other than the increased availability of home and community-based services and the decreased availability of informal care. Clearly, utilization is influenced by factors other than simply a need for care and the access to care. The contribution of social factors in explaining or predicting utilization rates renders projected estimates of cost almost impossible. Current projections of demand for formal long-term care (Rivlin & Wiener, 1988; Spillman & Kemper, 1992; Stone & Murtaugh, 1990) probably represent upper bounds not likely to be experienced.

ENDNOTE

1. The Hosmer-Lemeshow goodness-of-fit statistic compares observed and expected values in 10 subgroups of equal size, defined on the basis of the deciles of the predicted values from the fitted model (Hosmer & Lemeshow, 1989; Hosmer, Taber, & Lemeshow, 1991).

REFERENCES

AARP. (1993). *Reforming the health care system: State profiles, 1993*. Washington, DC: American Association of Retired Persons.

Administration on Aging (1994). *Infrastructure of home and community based services for the functionally impaired elderly*. Washington DC: U.S. Department of Health and Human Services.

Doty, P. (1986). Family care of the elderly: The role of public policy. *Milbank Quarterly*, *64*(1), 34-75.

Evashwick, C., Rowe, G., Diehr, P., & Branch, L. (1984). Factors explaining the use of health care services by the elderly. *Health Services Research*, *19*(3), 357-382.

Hanley, R. J., Wiener, J. M., & Harris, K. M. (1991). Will paid home care erode informal support? *Journal of Health Politics, Policy and Law*, *16*, 507-21.

Harrow, B., Tennstedt, S., & McKinlay, J. (in press). How costly is it to care for the disabled elderly in a community setting? *The Gerontologist*.

Horowitz, A. (1985). Family caregiving to the frail elderly. In N. P. Lawton & G. Maddox (eds.), *Annual Review of Gerontology and Geriatrics* (pp. 194-246). New York: Springer Publishing Company.

Hosmer, D. W., & Lemeshow, S. (1989). *Applied logistic regression*. New York: Wiley.

Hosmer, D. W., Taber, S., & Lemeshow, S. (1991). The importance of assessing the fit of logistic regression models: A case study. *American Journal of Public Health*, *81*, 1630-1635.

Hu, T-W., Huang, L.-F., & Cartwright, W. S. (1986). Evaluation of the costs of caring for the senile demented elderly: A pilot study. *The Gerontologist*, *26*, 158-163.

Kemper, P. (1992). The use of formal and informal home care by the disabled elderly. *Health Services Research*, *27* (4), 421-451.

Leon, J., & Lair, T. (1990). Functional status of the noninstitutionalized elderly: estimates of ADL and IADL difficulties. In *National Medical Expenditure Survey Research Findings 4*. Washington DC: US Department of Health and Human Services, National Center for Health Services Research.

Liang, K. Y., & Zeger, S. L. (1986). Longitudinal data analysis using generalized linear models. *Biometrika*, *73*, 13-22.

Lipsitz, S. R., & Harrington, D. P. (1990). Analyzing correlated binary data using SAS. *Computers and Biomedical Research*, *23*, 268-282.

Liu, K., Manton, K. G., & Liu, B. M. (1985). Home care expenses for the disabled elderly. *Home Care Financing Review*, *7*, 51-58.

Macken, C. (1986). A profile of the functionally impaired elderly persons living in the community. *Health Care Financing Review*, *7*, 33-49.

Max, W., Webber, P., & Fox, P. (1995). Alzheimer's disease: The unpaid burden of caregiving. *Journal of Aging and Health*, *7* (2), 179-199.

McAuley, W. J., & Arling, G. (1984). Use of in-home care by very old people. *Journal of Health and Social Behavior*, *25*(4), 54-64.

McKinlay, J., & Tennstedt, S. (1986). *Social Networks and the Care of Frail Elders: Final Report to the National Institute on Aging*. Final Report to the National Institute on Aging, Grant No. AG3869. Boston: Boston University.
National Academy on Aging (1994). *Old age in the 21st century*. Syracuse, NY: Syracuse University.
Noelker, L. S., & Wallace, R. W. (1985). The organization of family care for impaired elderly. *Journal of Family Issues*, *6* (1), 23-44.
Rice, D., Fox, P., Webber, P., Lindeman, D., Hauck, W., & Segura, E. (1993). The economic burden of Alzheimer's disease. *Health Affairs (Summer)*, 164-176.
Rivlin, A. M., & Wiener, J. M. (1988). *Caring for the disabled elderly*. Washington, DC: The Brookings Institution.
Shanas, E., Townsend, P., Wedderburn, D., Friis, H., Milhoj, P., & Stehouwer, J. (1968). *Old people in three industrial societies*. New York: Atherton.
Soldo, B. J., Agree, E., & Wolf, D. (1989). Balance between formal and informal care. In M. Ory & K. Bond (Eds.), *Aging and health care* (pp. 193-216). New York: Routledge.
Soldo, B. J., Wolf, D, & Agree, E. (1990). Family, households, and care arrangements of frail older women: A structural analysis. *The Journals of Gerontology, 45*(6), S238-S249.
Spillman, B., & Kemper, P. (1992). Long term care arrangements for elderly persons with disabilities: private and public roles. *Home Health Care Services Quarterly, 12*(1/2), 5-34.
Stone, R. I., & Kemper, P. (1989). Spouses and children of disabled elders: How large a constituency for long-term care reform? *Milbank Quarterly, 67* (3-4), 485-506.
Stone, R. I., & Murtaugh, C. M. (1990). The elderly population with chronic functional disability: Implications for home care eligibility. *The Gerontologist*, *30*, 491-96.
Sussman, M. (1979). Social and economic supports and family environments for the elderly. In *Final Report to the Administration on Aging*, Grant #90-A-316(03).
Tennstedt, S., Crawford, S., & McKinlay, J. (1993). Is family care on the decline? A longitudinal investigation of the substitution of long-term care services for informal care. *Milbank Memorial Quarterly*, 7 (4), 601-624.
Tennstedt, S. L., Sullivan, L. M., McKinlay, J. B., & D'Agostino, R. B. (1990). How important is functional status as a predictor of service use by older people? *Journal of Aging and Health*, *2*(4), 439-461.
U. S. Bureau of Labor Statistics (1993). Table 5: Median weekly earnings of wage and salary workers who usually work full time, by detailed occupation, 1983-91 annual wages. Data derived from Current Population Surveys.
U. S. Department of Commerce, Bureau of the Census (1992). Table 692, "Average Annual Income and Expenditure of all Consumer Units: 1990." In *Statistical Abstract of the United States: 1992* (pp. 442-443). Washington, DC.
U. S. General Accounting Office (1988). *Long-term care for the elderly: Issues of need, access and cost*. Washington, DC.
Wan, T. T. H., & Arling, G. (1983). Differential use of health services among disabled elderly. *Research on Aging*, *5*, 411-432.

Race and Gender Differences in the Distribution of Home and Community-Based Services in Florida

Lein Han, PhD

Health Care Financing Administration
Boston, Massachusetts

Charles Barrilleaux, PhD
Jill Quadagno, PhD

Florida State University

SUMMARY. This article examines the distribution of home and community-based services (HCBS) under Florida's Medicaid waiver program. Controlling for personal and community characteristics, it was found that gender and race significantly affect the access of the disabled adult population to HCBS services, with women and nonwhites significantly more likely to be receiving HCBS services. At the county level, the likelihood of one's being in the waiver program is contingent on the racial composition and level of segregation of the county. People residing in counties with substantial proportions of nonwhites are less likely to receive HCBS services–whatever

---

Lein Han is a statistician with the Division of Health Standards and Quality, Health Care Financing Administration, Region I, Boston, MA. Charles Barrilleaux is Associate Professor of Political Science and a member of the Policy Sciences Center faculty at Florida State University. Jill Quadagno, an Editor for this volume, is Mildred and Claude Pepper Eminent Scholar in Social Geronotology, Florida State University, with the Pepper Institute on Aging and Public Policy, Tallahassee, FL 32306.

[Haworth co-indexing entry note]: "Race and Gender Differences in the Distribution of Home and Community-Based Services in Florida." Han, Lein, Charles Barrilleaux, and Jill Quadagno. Co-published simultaneously in *Journal of Aging & Social Policy* (The Haworth Press, Inc.) Vol. 7, No. 3/4, 1996, pp. 93-107; and: *From Nursing Homes to Home Care* (ed: Marie E. Cowart and Jill Quadagno) The Haworth Press, Inc., 1996, pp. 93-107. Single or multiple copies of this article are available from The Haworth Document Delivery Service [1-800-342-9678, 9:00 a.m. - 5:00 p.m. (EST)].

their race. However, the higher the rate of racial segregation in the county, the higher the probability that the Medicaid disabled adult population will receive HCBS services. The Medicaid waiver program allows older, disabled black women to remain in their home neighborhoods rather than having to move to predominantly white areas where nursing homes are concentrated. Thus, the HCBS program not only provides them with a form of care that is preferred by most older people but also resolves market problems stemming from the lack of nursing homes in segregated areas by taking advantage of support systems in black households. *[Article copies available from The Haworth Document Delivery Service: 1-800-342-9678.]*

The largest public source of spending for long-term care services is through the Medicaid program. Medicaid-financed home and community-based (HCBS) services are provided to older persons and to disabled younger persons through mandatory Medicaid state services, through election of one or more optional benefits in the Medicaid plan, and through home and community-based waiver programs (Folkemer, 1994). Despite the availability of such options, approximately 85% of Medicaid long-term care spending is for institutional services compared to only 15% for HCBS services (National Academy on Aging, 1994). Nationwide, however, HCBS expenditures are expanding. Between 1991 and 1993 total spending for Medicaid HCBS services increased by 20.4% from $4.8 billion to $5.7 billion (Folkemer, 1994).

The implementation of HCBS programs raises a number of questions. What type of services are provided? Are the services adequate to meet the needs of the disabled? And are the services distributed according to rational and fair criteria? As Joshua Wiener and Raymond Hanley (1992, p. 78) note, "One major barrier to the expansion of . . . home care benefits is the lack of information on the determinants of home care use. . . . Information on who uses home care and how much they use, as well as on the dynamics affecting these choices is critical to designing public and private programs and estimating their potential costs."

One commonly used criterion for determining access to home care services is some measure of activities of daily living (ADLs), which indicates an individual's ability to function in the community. ADLs include problems with bathing, dressing, toileting, and so forth. A second criterion is cognitive impairment (Wiener & Hanley, 1992). The question, however, is whether rational criteria based on health and functioning are uniformly applied or whether other informal factors also affect eligibility for given programs. Existing research indicates no consistent relationship between individual attributes like age, gender, or race and the use of home care services (Wiener & Hanley, 1992). Part of the difficulty is that these studies do not necessarily examine similar programs. Some are concerned with private-pay home care, while others focus on pubic programs. There is some research on the Medicaid program indicating that various biases are present in the distribution of services. Madonna Meyer (1994), for example, finds that African Americans, women and nonmarried persons are not only more likely to be eligible for Medicaid in nursing homes but also more likely to be Medicaid-eligible upon admission than white, married men. Lein Han (1994) also finds variations in access to services in the Project AIDS Care program in Florida, a home and community-based services program for persons with HIV/AIDS. Han's research shows that although black males are disproportionately represented among those with the HIV/AIDS virus, white males are more likely to receive services through the HCBS program. This article reports on an examination of the distribution of HCBS services in Florida through the state's Medicaid waiver program.

THE MEDICAID WAIVER PROGRAM

In response to concerns among state legislatures that the Medicaid program was encouraging costly and unnecessary institutionalization of the disabled elderly, the Omnibus Budget Reconciliation Act of 1981 allowed states to apply for waivers that permit Medicaid to pay for non-medical community-based services for those who might be able to avoid institutionalization. The Home and Community-Based Waiver Services Program under Section 1915c of the Social Security Act allows states to offer a variety of supportive services. However, the total cost of the HCBS program must not exceed expenditures for institutional care that would have been incurred for these individuals in the absence of a waiver. Because of this regulation, a ceiling exists on the number of waiver slots available to a state (Neuschler, 1987).

Although states have certain services that must be included in their Medicaid plans, they also have broad discretion in selecting and defining the other services to be offered. Section 1915c also allows states to define geographic areas and target populations to be served. Thus, states have flexibility in determining where they provide services and who will receive these services. As of July 1, 1993, 45 states had 1915c waivers that provided HCBS services to the disabled (Folkemer, 1994).

Florida's 1915c program is administered by the Department of Elder Affairs. Preadmission screening is conducted through the Comprehensive Assessment and Review for Long Term Care Services program (CARES). This screening is required under federal law regarding Medicaid for those seeking nursing home care and includes functional, psychological and medical data to determine if an individual can remain in the community with appropriate formal and informal supports (Polivka, Dunlop, & Rothman, 1993).

According to waiver regulations, an individual is eligible if he or she would be likely to require care in a nursing home but for the provision of HCBS services. The financial eligibility requirements are mandated and must be identical to the requirements for Medicaid eligibility for nursing home care. In Florida for 1993, the income limit for Medicaid eligibility for nursing home care was set at 300% of SSI and the asset limit at $2,000.

In regard to other eligibility criteria, however, the state has considerable discretion. This is especially true in evaluating the applicant's support system. The assessment instrument asks a series of questions under the category "client support" regarding the amount of help the individual receives for personal care assistance, housekeeping, transportation, shopping, personal finances, services from a health professional, adult day care, and home-delivered meals. The instrument also asks who provides the help, the frequency of help, and the amount of additional help needed. A second group of questions examines "social resources," including whether the client lives alone, the availability of kin to stay with the client if necessary, and the presence of a support network as measured by the individual having someone to talk to about problems, number of times per week he or she spends talking on the phone to friends and relatives, and amount of visits with friends and relatives. The qualitative nature of these factors provides the caseworker with considerable discretion in determining who might be eligible for HCBS services.

METHOD AND DATA ANALYSIS

Description of the Population

A study to analyze the distribution of home and community-based services under Florida's Medicaid waiver program was conducted by the authors in 1993. The study population consisted of 54,120 Medicaid beneficiaries between the ages of 20 and 115 who were reimbursed for at least one claim between July 1, 1992 and June 30, 1993 for the following categories of services: (1) skilled nursing home, (2) intermediate level care I, and (3) intermediate level care II, or for (4) the Aged and Disabled Waiver Program (ADA) for HCBS.[1] Recipients whose county of residence was miscoded or missing from the Medicaid eligibility file were excluded.

The respondents included 48,398 Medicaid adult recipients who were functionally disabled and receiving nursing home care and 5,722 who had received at least one ADA community-based service during the study period. As Table 1 shows, the average age of the subjects was 81. There are race and gender differences in average age, with females being slightly older (82) than males (76) and whites older (82) than nonwhites (77). Those receiving ADA HCBS services were younger (75) than those in institutional care (82).

Women and nonwhites were disproportionately represented in the ADA HCBS program. Women comprise 70% of the eligible Medicaid beneficiaries but 80% of the ADA HCBS recipients. Similarly, nonwhites comprise 16% of the study population but 29% of ADA HCBS recipients.

Personal characteristics were extracted from the Medicaid eligibility and claims data files. Community characteristics were compiled from the 1990 federal census report and the Medicaid provider files.

Hypotheses

Existing research on the use of health services typically draws upon personal and community characteristics as influences on the use of services. Our model of participation in the home and community-based services (HCBS) program used here is based roughly on the model of access to health services developed originally by Ronald Anderson and James Newman (1973). Anderson and Newman's conceptual model identified three sources of variations in individual use of health services–personal attributes, the availability of services, and the social setting within which the services are delivered.

In addition to these, the effect of a fourth factor that is less readily measurable–the structure of the program–is discussed. Program structure includes the nature of the process for determining eligibility and the eligibility rules themselves.

It is assumed that personal and community characteristics affect the likelihood of an individual's being enrolled in the Medicaid HCBS program. Personal attributes or characteristics include age, race, gender, the number of months the individual was enrolled in an HMO, and the number of inpatient hospital days and/or nursing home days for which claims or payments were made in the previous year. These individual-level variables were then expressed in the hypotheses below:

- H_1 Whites are less likely to use HCBS services than non-whites.
- H_2 Women are more likely to use HCBS services than men.
- H_3 Longer HMO enrollments are expected to increase the likelihood of HCBS enrollment.

H_4 Older persons are less apt to be enrolled in HCBS programs.
H_5 The higher the number of inpatient hospital days, the lower the HCBS enrollment.
H_6 The higher the number of nursing home days, the lower the HCBS enrollment.

The expectation that elderly whites are less likely to use HCBS as a method of care is derived from differences in the organization of white and nonwhite households. As Table 2 shows, while there is little difference between black and white older women in the percentage living alone, older black women are much more likely to be living with other relatives (41% of blacks 75 and older compared to 19% of whites). These patterns of household composition support research which demonstrates that among blacks, adult children are frequent providers of assistance to their parents (Chatters & Taylor, 1993). Other factors that might reduce the likelihood of whites in the HCBS program include the higher residential mobility of whites and the easier access to institutional care for elders enjoyed by whites. In addition, nonwhites are more apt than whites to seek services in settings other than private offices or other mainstream institutions (Dutton, 1978). Thus, we expect nonwhites (African Americans, in this subset of the Medicaid population) to rely more heavily upon HCBS. Given this, we can also expect a negative relationship between this measure of race, in which "white" is coded 1 and other races are coded 0.

Men would be less likely to receive services via HCBS than women, because of their income and household arrangements. As Table 2 shows, white men are most likely to be living with a spouse (70% of those 75 and older), whereas black women are least likely to be living with a spouse (14% of those 75 and older). Living with a spouse will affect HCBS services in two ways, according to our hypotheses. First, men living with a spouse may be less likely than individuals in other household arrangements to apply for HCBS services. This is partly because married men have the highest incomes among the elderly. White, married couples over 65 have a median income of $24,616 compared to $5,962 for single, black women (Grad, 1994). Thus, married men are most able to pay privately for home care services. Their higher incomes would also make them ineligible for Medicaid. A second factor, that can't be measured, is that married men living with a spouse may be viewed by caseworkers who screen applicants as less in need of services.

Men also can be considered less likely to be receiving HCBS services because of population characteristics. The elderly Medicaid population is comprised mainly of widowed women; many of them attained Medicaid eligibility only after spending down their assets in caring for a spouse,

TABLE 1. Simple Statistics for Explanatory Variables

Variable	Mean	Standard Deviation	Minimum	Maximum
Race	0.82	0.38	0.00	1.00
Sex	0.25	0.43	0.00	1.00
HMO months	0.02	0.49	0.00	12.00
Age	81.06	12.001	21.00	112.00
Inpatient hospital days	0.50	3.83	0.00	45.00
Nursing home days	53.89	110.61	0.00	487.00
HCBS provider/ ADA population	1.44	0.98	0.21	20.41
Nursing home beds/ADA population	444.74	247.72	0.00	1311.88
Doctors/county population	0.61	0.23	0.00	1.69
Medicaid doctors/ recipients	6.13	1.70	0.43	23.26
Hospital beds ratio	5.41	4.13	0.00	50.07
Metropolitan	0.87	0.34	0.00	1.00
Median family income	31.88	4.08	20.54	40.73
Nonwhite population county	16.56	8.05	3.00	59.00
Segregation rate	52.50	11.33	2.00	71.00

TABLE 2. Household Composition by Race and Gender Among Persons Sixty-Five and Older

	White Persons (Percent Living)			Black Persons (Percent Living)		
	Alone	With Spouse	With Other Relatives	Alone	With Spouse	With Other Relatives
Male						
65 and older	15	76	6	30	54	12
65-74	12	79	6	28	58	9
75 and older	21	70	7	32	46	17
Female						
65 and older	42	41	14	40	25	33
65-74	34	54	11	39	32	28
75 and older	53	25	19	43	14	41

Source: U.S. Bureau of the Census, 1993, p. 20-468.

who may have died as the family resources were being depleted. It is hypothesized that enrollment in an HMO will be related positively to the likelihood of being enrolled in an HCBS. Months of enrollment in an HMO capture an individual's preferences for insurance coverage and the length of his or her coverage under a capitated plan.[2] Longer durations in a capitated plan are presumed to be linked to enrollment in HCBS. The likelihood of being enrolled in the HCBS program would diminish with increased age, with older persons more in need of institutional care. The likelihood of using HCBS would diminish along with increased use of hospital inpatient services and/or increased claims for nursing home reimbursements. In either case, individual use of institutional services acts as a direct substitute for HCBS.

Community-level determinants of participation in HCBS include measures of availability of HCBS providers in a county, the supply of nursing home beds, the supply of physicians, the rate of physician participation in Medicaid, the supply of hospital beds, the metropolitan character of the county (or lack of it), the nonwhite percentage of a county's population, and the rate of residential segregation. Regarding community-level influences, these were the hypotheses arrived upon. The likelihood of HCBS being used:

H_7 is *higher* where the supply of HCBS providers is higher.
H_8 is *lower* where the supply of nursing home beds is higher.
H_9 is *lower* where the supply of physicians is higher.
H_{10} is *higher* where physician participation in Medicaid is higher.
H_{11} is *higher* where the supply of hospital beds is higher.

H_{12} is *higher* in metropolitan areas.
H_{13} is *lower* where median family incomes are lower.
H_{14} is *lower* where the percentage of the nonwhite population is higher.
H_{15} is *higher* where the rate of residential segregation is higher.

The "supply of services" hypotheses (H_7-H_{11}) capture characteristics of local service markets expected to influence the ability of individuals to participate in HCBS. Generally, it was assumed that market characteristics would reflect the prevailing organization of medical services in a given county, and the use of services would result directly from that organization. Since data for this study were organized cross-sectionally, only speculative comment can be made on the temporal order by which supply relationships are established. A greater supply–therefore availability–of HCBS providers would indicate more use of the services. Likewise, more nursing home beds would be associated with lower use of HCBS, since HCBS use is a direct competitor with nursing homes; a *better* well-established nursing home sector would likely introduce competition for enrollments in HCBS and diminish participation in HCBS. HCBS enrollments are expected to be lower where there are more physicians in an area, but higher where larger proportions of physicians participate in Medicaid. Finally, HCBS participation would increase where there are more hospital beds because hospitals should seek to expand into HCBS to compete with nursing homes for that segment of the Medicaid market.

Other county-level characteristics that could have some influence on an individual's likelihood of using HCBS include whether or not an individual lives within a metropolitan area,[3] median family income in the individual's county of residence, the percentage of the nonwhite population in the county within which an individual lives, and the degree to which the Medicaid enrollee's county of residence is racially segregated. Eligible persons living in metropolitan areas as defined here would be more likely to make use of HCBS, largely because of the scale economies for the program available as opposed to that for rural areas. We expect individuals living in counties with relatively higher median family incomes to be less likely to use HCBS, since higher income persons are more likely to have family resources upon which to draw; they also may prove more likely to receive care in institutional settings. The likelihood of enrollment in HCBS would diminish in areas where the nonwhite population is greater; where there are large numbers of nonwhites in the population, there are likely also to be better developed institutionally based services. Finally, people are more likely to rely upon HCBS in areas that have higher levels of residential segregation.

To summarize, a mixture of personal and county level characteristics of a certain type would help predict which individuals would enroll in HCBS. Our model is estimated using the logistic regression routine included in SAS mainframe software.

Results

Logistic regression results are reported in Table 3. The dependent variable for the analysis is a binary indicator coded 1 for individuals who are enrolled in the Home and Community Based Services program, and 0 otherwise. The estimates provide support for the majority of our hypotheses, all of which have signs in the expected direction and the majority of which attain statistical significance.

Among the personal characteristics expected to influence the likelihood of using HCBS, whites' probability of receiving HCBS was .91 less than that of nonwhites in our sample, and women were .70 less likely than men to do so. Each additional month spent enrolled in an HMO increased the likelihood of receiving HCBS by .23, and each added year of age reduced

TABLE 3. Logit Analysis of Access to ADA HCBS Program

Variable	Parameter Estimate
Intercept	3**
Personal Characteristics	
Race (white = 1)	−0.91**
Sex (male = 1)	−0.70**
HMO months	0.23**
Age	−0.05**
Inpatient hospital days	−0.03**
Nursing home days	−0.02
Community Characteristics	
HCBS provider/ADA population	0.29**
NH beds/ADA population	−0.002**
Doctors/County population	−0.07
Medicaid Doc./Recipients	0.02
Hospital beds/County population	0.01**
Metropolitan	0.20
Median family income	−0.01*
Nonwhite population (%)	−0.01**
Segregation rate	0.001**

ADA: Florida Medicaid Aged and Disabled Adult Waiver
HCBS: Home and Community-Based Services
*probability ≤ .01
**probability ≤ .05

the likelihood of HCBS by .05. Likewise, each added day spent as an inpatient in a hospital lessened the likelihood of receiving HCBS by .02. Nursing home days had no significant effect on the likelihood of receiving HCBS.

Among the community characteristics effects that were tested, the supply of HCBS providers has a statistically significant positive influence on the likelihood that an individual will receive HCBS: each one-unit increase in the ratio of HCBS providers to the ADA population increases the likelihood of receiving HCBS services by .29. A weaker negative effect is seen with the supply of nursing home beds: a one-unit increase in the ratio of nursing home beds to ADA population results in a .002 decrease in the likelihood that a person will receive HCBS. The supply of physicians or Medicaid physicians had no significant effect on the likelihood of using HCBS, while the supply of hospital beds increased the likelihood of receiving HCBS by a small amount (.01). Finally, each dollar decline in median family income decreased the likelihood of using HCBS by .01, and each percentage increase in nonwhite population similarly reduced the likelihood of HCBS. Finally, each one-unit increase of residential segregation increased the likelihood that an individual would receive HCBS by .001.

DISCUSSION

Evidence from the study reported on here suggests significant racial and gender differences in the use of HCBS. Thus, there are nontrivial differences in how portions of the eligible population respond to the opportunity to receive support in the home and community versus in an institution. The study's results suggest that, as in other attempts to modify the delivery of health services, personal and environmental characteristics exert important influences on program outcomes. The finding that nonwhites and women are more likely to receive HCBS than whites and men suggests that HCBS represents a "nontraditional" venue for receipt of services. Nonwhites often avoid the receipt of services in private offices or other mainstream institutions partly because they feel some psychological and social discomfort in doing so (Dutton, 1978). "Mainstream" settings are cast as reflecting middle-class orientations and values, which may introduce some discomfort for persons whose upbringings differ, leading them to seek services in other venues. These results may reflect that discomfort, but they may also indicate, at least in the case of nonwhites, the presence of a better system of home support than is in place in the white community. Because the decision to place persons in the home-based system is made largely by caseworkers, information on their decisionmaking process would be a valuable source for further insights about the factors that influence determinations.

Although the data do not address the characteristics of living situations, and so forth, we can speculate that nonwhite households may be more likely to have a supportive family network than white households; one might reasonably expect that the value of an extended-family support network is felt at both ends of the life cycle. African-American households, though more likely than white households to be female-headed, are also more likely than white households to have members other than the nuclear family. That is, elders are helpful for parents with young children and may provide essential support for parents, particularly in low-income households, and younger family members may continue to be important caregivers for the ADA population in the nonwhite community. Whites may be more likely to qualify for Medicaid through its spenddown provisions and so may be more apt to need institutionalized care than nonwhites at the point where they are counted among the ADA Medicaid population.

Also related to race, the results of the study are interesting. Data suggest that enrollment in HCBS lessens as the percentage of nonwhite population increases, but use of HCBS increases as residential segregation rises. These results point to a complicated relationship between the variables. For example, nursing home beds in Florida are clustered in more affluent counties. Having held constant the effects of metropolitan residential location and income, there is a negative influence of the percentage of the nonwhite population participating in HCBS. These findings suggest that areas with higher nonwhite populations reduce HCBS participation. However, the study results suggest also that nonwhites are more likely to participate in HCBS than whites; this is likely attributable to the segregation-rate variable. The results and ancillary analyses suggest that nursing homes are essentially clustered in areas where relatively affluent elderly live, the majority of whom are white (remember that whites are less apt to use HCBS). The segregation-rate variable may be capturing what amounts to de facto segregation in nursing homes in Florida: areas that are heavily black are not especially lucrative places in which to establish nursing homes, the essence of HCBS is to allow the client to remain in the community from which he or she comes, and HCBS thus allows nonwhite members of the ADA population to receive services in the segregated areas in which they live.

The coefficients that capture the supply of HCBS providers and the supply of nursing home beds suggest that, consistent with existing research on Medicaid innovations, the market appears to drive what services individuals receive. Charles Barrilleaux and Mark Miller (1992) report market characteristics–the supply of physicians and hospital beds–and the amount paid for physician visits to be the strongest determinants of access to care for individuals in state Medicaid programs. The study results suggest that where nursing home beds are available the use of HCBS is lower. Thus, HCBS appears to be a substitute for nursing home care where such care is not available rather than the competitor it is designed, at least partly, to be. This may have implications for cost-control efforts, particularly in an age in which various forms of managed care are being proposed as solutions to the problems of high spending, poor access to services, and so on. This is related to the argument concerning the effects of residential segregation: some areas may be potentially lucrative for the establishment of nursing homes but other areas are not so attractive. HCBS flourishes in the least attractive market areas. As a result, as with clinics and hospital outpatient departments, which are frequented disproportionately by nonwhite Medicaid recipients (Long, Settle, & Stuart, 1986), HCBS may provide needed services in the nonwhite community.

CONCLUSION

The states have considerable flexibility in determining who will receive home care services through their Medicaid waiver programs, and where these services will be concentrated. Ideally, this flexibility allows states to tailor services to fit the needs of the population. The implementation of the Medicaid waiver program in Florida has operated in precisely this fashion. The program disproportionately serves the nonwhite population in areas where institutional care is least available. The question is whether the distribution of these services, which are concentrated in racially segregated communities, circumvents Medicaid's stated goal of providing individuals' access to "mainstream" care. The data to answer this question directly is not available, but indirect evidence allows us to speculate about the consequences of the findings of this study.

In some respects, the Medicaid waiver program may inadvertently reinforce racial segregation of older, disabled minorities by allowing them to remain in their home neighborhoods rather than moving to predominantly white areas where nursing homes are concentrated. It also, however, provides older blacks, especially black women, with a form of care that is preferred by most older people. As implemented, the HCBS program appears to resolve market problems stemming from the lack of nursing homes in segregated areas by taking advantage of support systems in African American households.

If the interpretation of the study reported on here is accurate, then the Medicaid waiver program is likely to have little impact on reducing the demand for nursing home care. Rather than providing an alternative to institutionalization, it serves as a substitute. The wider implications of this conclusion are that if other Medicaid waiver programs operate similarly, they will have little effect in reducing Medicaid costs. Rather, these programs appear to establish two separate systems of care for the disabled elderly, those who are not served by the more conventional venues.

ENDNOTES

1. Skilled nursing homes, intermediate level care facilities I, and intermediate level care facilities II are clustered according to the intensity of care delivered, with skilled facilities providing the most intensive services, intermediate level care facilities I providing services of an intensity a step below that, and intermediate care facilities III providing the least medically intensive services. Assignment of individuals to the Aged and Disabled Waiver Program is based on case worker interpretations of their health needs and available social support and, at least in theory, a person in any of the three aforementioned service needs categories could be placed in the waiver program.

2. Capitated plans are those in which the costs of an enrollee's care are prepaid based on some agreed-upon pricing structure and are contrasted with fee-for-service plans.

3. Using the Census Bureau's current definition, which requires that the area have a city with at least 50,000 population or a recognized urban area of at least 50,000 within a broader area with population of not less than 100,000.

REFERENCES

Anderson, R., & Newman, J. (1973). Societal and individual determinants of medical care utilization in the United States. *Milbank Memorial Fund Quarterly, 51*, 95-124.

Barrilleaux, C. J., & Miller, M. (1992). Decisions without consequences: Cost control and access in state Medicaid programs. *Journal of Health Politics, Policy and Law, 17*, 97-118.

Chatters, L., & Taylor, R. (1993). Intergenerational support: The provision of assistance to parents by adult children. In J. S. Jackson, L. M. Chatters, & R. J. Taylor (Eds.), *Aging in Black America* (pp. 69-83). Newbury Park, CA: Sage.

Dutton, D. (1978). Explaining the low use of health services by the poor: Cost, attitudes, or service delivery systems? *American Sociological Review, 48*, 348-68.

Folkemer, D. (1994). State use of home and community-based services for the aged under Medicaid: Waiver programs, personal care, frail elderly services and home health services. #9405 AARP Public Policy Institute. Washington, DC: American Association of Retired Persons.

Grad, S. (1994). *Income of the population 55 or older, 1992*. Social Security Administration, Office of Research and Statistics, SSA Publications No 13-11871.

Han, L. (1994). *Gender, race and access to health care: Florida Medicaid and AIDS*. Unpublished doctoral dissertation. Tallahassee, FL: Florida State University.

Long, S. H., Settle, R., & Stuart, B. (1986). Reimbursement and access to physicians' services under Medicaid. *Journal of Health Economics*, *5*, 235-51.

Meyer, M. H. (1994). Institutional bias and Medicaid use in nursing homes. *Journal of Aging Studies*, *8* (2), 179-194.

National Academy on Aging. (1994). Old age in the 21st century. A report to the Assistant Secretary for Aging. U.S. Dept. of Health and Human Services.

Neuschler, E. (1987). *Medicaid eligibility for the elderly in need of long term care*. Washington, DC: National Governor's Association.

Polivka, L., Dunlop, B., & Rothman, M. (1993). *Long-term care in Florida: A policy framework for expanding community programs and increasing administrative and service delivery efficiency*. Florida Policy Exchange Center on Aging. Tampa, FL: University of South Florida.

U.S. Bureau of the Census. (1993). *Current population reports*. Washington, DC: U.S. Government Printing Office.

Wiener, J. M., & Hanley, R. J. (1992). Caring for the disabled elderly: There's no place like home. In S. M. Shortell & U. Reinhart (Eds.), *Improving health policy and management* (pp. 75-109). Ann Arbor, MI: Health Administration Press.

Financing Reform for Long-Term Care: Strategies for Public and Private Long-Term Care Insurance

Joshua M. Wiener, PhD

The Brookings Institution
Washington, DC

SUMMARY. The way the nation provides for the financing and delivery of long-term care is badly in need of reform. The principal options for change are private insurance, altering Medicaid, and

Joshua M. Wiener is a Senior Fellow at the Brookings Institution, where he specializes in health policy.

The opinions in this article are those of the author and do not necessarily represent the views of other staff members, officers, or trustees of the Brookings Institution.

The author can be contacted at: The Brookings Institution, 1775 Massachusetts Avenue, NW, Washington, DC 20036.

[Haworth co-indexing entry note]: "Financing Reform for Long-Term Care: Strategies for Public and Private Long-Term Care Insurance." Wiener, Joshua M. Co-published simultaneously in *Journal of Aging & Social Policy* (The Haworth Press, Inc.) Vol. 7, No. 3/4, 1996, pp. 109-127; and: *From Nursing Homes to Home Care* (ed: Marie E. Cowart and Jill Quadagno) The Haworth Press, Inc., 1996, pp. 109-127. Single or multiple copies of this article are available from The Haworth Document Delivery Service [1-800-342-9678, 9:00 a.m. - 5:00 p.m. (EST)].

public long-term care insurance. This article uses the Brookings-ICF Long-Term Care Financing Model to evaluate each of these options in terms of affordability, distribution of benefits, and ability to reduce catastrophic out-of-pocket costs. So long as private insurance is aimed at the elderly, its market penetration and ability to finance long-term care will remain severely limited. Affordability is a major problem. Selling to younger persons could solve the affordability problem, but marketing is extremely difficult. Liberalizing Medicaid could help solve the problems of long-term care, but there is little public support for means-tested programs. Finally, universalistic public insurance programs do well in meeting the goals of long-term care reform, but all social insurance programs are expensive and seem politically infeasible in the current political environment.
[Article copies available from The Haworth Document Delivery Service: 1-800-342-9678.]

The way the nation provides for the financing and delivery of long-term care is badly in need of reform. No other part of the health care system generates as much passionate discontent as does long-term care. At the heart of the problem is the absence of any satisfactory way to help people anticipate and pay for long-term care. The disabled elderly find, often to their surprise, that the costs of nursing home and home care are not covered to any significant extent by Medicare or private insurance. Instead, they must rely on their own savings or, failing that, turn to welfare in the form of Medicaid. At a national average cost of $40,000 a year for nursing home care, long-term care is a leading cause of catastrophic out-of-pocket health care costs for the elderly. In addition, despite the strong preferences of the disabled for home and community-based services, current financing is highly skewed toward care in nursing homes.

While the debate over long-term care reform has many facets, it is primarily an argument over the relative merits of private- versus public-sector approaches. Differences over how much emphasis to put on each sector partly depend on values that cannot be directly proved or disproved. Some believe that the primary responsibility for care of the elderly belongs with individuals and their families, and that government should act only as a payer of last resort for those unable to provide for themselves. The opposite view is that the government should take the lead in ensuring comprehensive care for all disabled older people, regardless of financial need, by providing comprehensive, compulsory social insurance. In this view, there is little or no role for the private sector. Between these polar positions, many combinations of public and private responsibility are possible.

The choice of emphasis between public and private programs depends not just on political ideology, but also on whether private and public initiatives are affordable, whom they would benefit, and whether they can reduce catastrophic costs and realign the delivery system. For example, if it were demonstrably possible to market private long-term care insurance that would protect a large majority of the population from financial hardship and reduce dependence on Medicaid, then many people would see little need for new government programs. Conversely, if private insurance were not to prove widely affordable or to face other barriers that prevent people from voluntarily purchasing policies, then the case for an expanded public role would be stronger.

This article evaluates private insurance, public insurance, and Medicaid reform options for long-term care, primarily using the Brookings-ICF Long-Term Care Financing Model. Briefly, it seems likely that private insurance aimed at the elderly will grow, but remain a relatively small niche product. Affordability is a major barrier. Private insurance sold to the nonelderly population can largely solve those affordability problems, but faces daunting marketing barriers. All public-sector options do a better job than private-sector options in targeting expenditures to the elderly with more modest incomes and in reducing catastrophic out-of-pocket costs. However, all of the public-sector options, except for liberalization of the Medicaid program, require substantial increases in public spending. With the collapse of health care reform in 1994 and a sharply more conservative mood in Congress, expansions of public programs are highly unlikely, at least for the foreseeable future.

METHODS: THE BROOKINGS-ICF LONG-TERM CARE FINANCING MODEL

The Brookings-ICF Long-Term Care Financing Model is a large, integrated microsimulation model that projects the size, financial position, disability status, and nursing home and home care use and expenditures of the elderly through the year 2020. Details on the structure and assumptions of the model have been described elsewhere (Wiener, Illston, & Hanley, 1994). The model is designed to evaluate public- and private-sector options for long-term care financing reform.

Like all computer models, the Brookings-ICF Long-Term Care Financing Model embodies a large number of assumptions. Our mortality and economic assumptions generally follow those of the Social Security Administration actuaries' middle path. Thus, the model assumes that elderly mortality rates will continue to decline and that the economy, inflation, and wages will continue to grow at modest levels. In particular, real wages and fringe benefits are assumed to grow at 1.5% a year; general inflation is assumed to be 4.0% a year. Because of the large labor component of nursing home and home care, nursing home and home care prices are assumed to grow at 1.5% a year faster than general inflation. Although some recent analyses suggest that disability is declining among the elderly, disability rates are assumed to remain constant over time, as are nursing home and home care use rates (Manton, Corder, & Stallard, 1993).

BASE CASE: INCREASING STRAINS ON THE SYSTEM

As the population of disabled elderly increases, additional pressures on the long-term care financing system are inevitable. The "base case" simulates what may happen if there are no changes in the way long-term care services are organized, used, and reimbursed between 1993 and 2018. Alternative financing options are compared to what will happen under this benchmark scenario.

Over the next 25-year period, the number of elderly in this country will grow rapidly as will the use of and expenditures for nursing home and home care. Not surprisingly, then, the total number of elderly nursing home users during the course of one year is projected to increase from 2.2 million in 1993 to 3.6 million in 2018. Similarly, the number of home care users during the course of the year is projected to increase from 5.2 million to 7.4 million over the same period.

Nursing home and home care expenditures for the elderly will increase rapidly over the projected time period, from $54.7 billion in 1993 to $126.2 billion in constant 1993 dollars in 2018 (Table 1). Indeed, expenditures rise a good deal faster than use, primarily because nursing home and home care prices are likely to increase faster than general consumer prices. Despite projected improvements in the financial status of the elderly, the model projects Medicaid spending will increase nearly as fast as total long-term care expenditures.

A major concern of long-term care reform is to reduce out-of-pocket catastrophic costs, but there are many different ways to measure these financial burdens. Since Medicaid requires that nursing home patients spend down virtually all of their assets to contribute virtually all of their income to the cost of care, one measure of the extent of catastrophic costs is the number of Medicaid nursing home patients. The average annual number of elderly Medicaid nursing home patients is likely to increase from 1.4 million in 1993 to 2.0 million in 2018.

TABLE 1. Spending for Nursing Home and Home Care, Under Current Policies (Billions of 1993 Dollars)

Payment Source	1993	2018	Percentage Increase 1993 - 2018
Nursing Home Services			
Medicaid	$22.4	$49.0	118
Medicare	4.3	10.0	132
Out-of-Pocket	28.0	69.2	147
Total	**54.7**	**128.2**	**134**
Home Care Services			
Medicaid	3.6	5.2	45
Medicare	9.4	19.0	102
Other Payers	2.2	4.3	92
Out-of-Pocket	5.5	11.5	109
Total	**20.8**	**40.0**	**93**

Source: Brookings-ICF Long-Term Care Financing Model.

An alternate measure of catastrophic costs is to calculate the proportion of a patient's income and assets that are spent on nursing home care. The model projects that the proportion of nursing home admissions who will spend more than 40% of their income and financial assets on care will be fairly stable at about 40% of nursing home admissions during the simulation period.

PRIVATE LONG-TERM CARE INSURANCE

Private-sector approaches are appealing because they reflect the American tradition of individuals taking responsibility for their own lives. The classic virtue of the competitive market is that it has the flexibility to adapt to individual needs and wants and to local conditions. In the case of long-term care, the dream has been that private insurance could hold down public spending on Medicaid. The marked improvement in the financial position of the elderly in the past 20 years has also made it more plausible to argue that private insurance might be widely affordable in the future.

Although 97% of the elderly have Medicare coverage and almost two thirds have private insurance to supplement their Medicare coverage, insurance against the potentially devastating costs of long-term care is relatively rare and very recent. While the number of policies in force is considerably lower, the Health Insurance Association of America reports that the number of policies *ever sold* increased from 815,000 in 1987 to 2.9 million in 1993 (Coronel & Fulton, 1995). Thus, perhaps 4% to 5% of the elderly and a negligible percentage of the nonelderly have some kind of private long-term care insurance.

Individual Private Insurance Products

Private long-term care insurance is overwhelmingly sold on an individual, one-on-one basis to the elderly population, with the insured paying the entire cost of the premium. This is in contrast to acute care insurance, which is primarily provided through employment-based groups to the nonelderly where employers shoulder most of the cost.

Partly because of the high administrative costs and the relatively short period of time available for reserves to build, private long-term care insurance sold to the elderly is quite expensive. As a result, numerous studies conclude that only between 10% and 20% of the current elderly can afford high-quality private long-term care insurance (Friedland, 1990; Rivlin, Wiener, Spence, & Hanley, 1988; Zedlewski, Barnes, Burt, McBride, & Meyer, 1990).

Over the last few years, the substantial portion of American households that have life insurance policies has stimulated interest in using this mechanism–especially cash value policies that accumulate reserves–to finance long-term care. Since most nursing home patients end their stay because of death, insurers use "accelerated death benefits" to pay benefits a bit earlier than they would otherwise. The principal drawback of this approach is that many Americans do not have cash-value life insurance and most policies have only a small cash value. In 1991, the average face value of cash-value life insurance policies was only about $26,000 (American Council on Life Insurance, 1993). Since the cash value is small, policies cannot provide much in the way of long-term care coverage.

Strategies to Improve Affordability

In order to improve the affordability of private long-term care insurance, a variety of options have been proposed. These include encouraging people to buy insurance when they are still young and in the work force, providing tax deductions or tax credits for the purchase of insurance, and providing easier access to Medicaid for people who buy an approved long-term care policy.

Employer-sponsored policies. If people bought long-term care insurance when they were younger, especially through employer groups, then premiums could be significantly lower, and, therefore, more affordable. Policies bought at age 45, rather than age 65, have a longer time for reserves and interest earnings to build and group policies have lower administrative costs than policies sold individually. Although employer-sponsored policies are the fastest growing of all private insurance markets, only 400,000 such policies had been sold as of 1993 (Coronel & Fulton, 1995).

While conceptually sound, selling private long-term care insurance to an employer-based, younger population will be difficult. First, marketing will be extremely hard. In general, 45-year-old workers have other, more immediate concerns, such as child care, mortgage payments, and college education for their children. Experience to date is that few employees who are offered private long-term care insurance actually purchase it (Coronel & Fulton, 1995).

Second, selling to the nonelderly population raises several difficult pricing considerations. An actuary pricing a private long-term care insurance product for a 45-year-old must predict what is going to happen 40 years into the future, when the insured is 85 years old and likely to need services. Small changes in assumptions compounded over long periods of time can drastically change a product's profitability.

Closely related to the issue of pricing is the issue of product design. While employer-sponsored plans are sometimes better than the individually marketed products available, most policies do not deal well with the inevitable inflation in nursing home and home care.

Third, while employers may be willing to offer private long-term care insurance, they are unlikely to help pay for it as they do for acute care insurance. The uncertain tax status of employer contributions for private long-term care insurance undoubtedly complicates matters, but employers are not looking to contribute to another fringe benefit for retirees. It is no secret that acute care insurance premiums have skyrocketed and companies have been looking for ways to cut back on their expenses. In addition, large employers typically face huge unfunded liabilities for their acute care insurance for retirees.

Tax incentives for purchase of private long-term care insurance. Another set of options would improve the affordability of private long-term care insurance by offering a tax deduction or credit on federal income taxes to purchasers of private long-term care insurance. With either a deduction or a credit, the effect is to reduce the net price of insurance policies, making them more affordable. Some insurance advocates also argue that a tax incentive would send a signal to potential purchasers that the government considers long-term care insurance to be a worthwhile product.

Tax incentives are potentially inefficient because benefits are likely to go primarily to help people who would have bought the policies anyway. Thus, the government's cost per additional policy sold will be high.

In addition, a tax incentive is, by definition, a revenue loss that will increase the federal deficit unless offset by other revenue increases or spending cuts. Some advocates of tax incentives argue that the tax loss will be offset by reductions in Medicaid expenditures. For the level of incentives commonly suggested, our simulations suggest that this is not the case. At least through 2018, the tax loss will be at least four times the savings from public programs.

Easier access to Medicaid: A public-private partnership. A final option to promote private insurance has been to provide easier access to Medicaid for persons who purchase a state-approved private long-term care insurance policy. In these public-private partnerships, which are being tried in Connecticut, New York, Indiana, Iowa, and California, policyholders are allowed to keep more of their financial assets than is normally allowed and still receive Medicaid nursing home benefits. Under this strategy, it is possible to obtain lifetime asset protection without having to buy an insurance policy that pays lifetime benefits. Moreover, supporters argue that the scheme will be roughly budget-neutral in terms of government expenditures, with Medicaid savings offsetting the new benefits.

This approach raises several issues. First, is it appropriate to use Medicaid, a means-tested, welfare program, which is designed for the poorest of the poor, to protect the assets of primarily upper-middle and upper-income elderly?

Second, how important is "asset protection" as a motivator in the purchase of private long-term care insurance? In a 1990 survey of new long-term care insurance purchasers, LifePlans, Inc. found that while asset protection was one of many reasons people purchased insurance, only 14% of people buying coverage listed asset protection as the "most important" reason (Lifeplans, 1992).

The third concern is whether easier access to Medicaid will actually induce substantial numbers of people to purchase long-term care insurance who would not otherwise have bought it. Indeed, one of the major reasons people buy long-term care insurance is to avoid the need to apply for welfare, with its stigma, second-class access, and perhaps inadequate care. Proposed changes in the Medicaid program may accentuate this problem.

Private Insurance Simulation Results

Simulations using the Brookings-ICF Long-Term Care Financing Model show that private insurance for long-term care can grow substantially. Figure 1 summarizes the assumptions used for our simulations of the principal private insurance options, and Table 2 summarizes the results. These assumptions are relatively generous to the potential role of private long-term care insurance and are meant to establish a rough upper limit of the potential impact. They are not a prediction of what will happen.

The simulation results for private long-term care insurance suggest that the industry is at a crossroads. So long as private insurance is aimed principally at the elderly population, its market penetration and ability to finance long-term care will remain restricted, even 25 years into the future. Because of the limited market penetration, private insurance will not substantially reduce catastrophic out-of-pocket costs among the elderly. Moreover, private insurance expenditures will be made mostly on behalf of the upper-income elderly. As a result, private insurance sold to the elderly will have almost no impact on Medicaid expenditures.

The story changes substantially if employers could be convinced to offer private long-term care insurance to their active employees, and if workers were willing to buy the policies. The simulation results clearly suggest that the affordability problem of long-term care insurance can largely be solved by selling properly structured policies to the nonelderly. Indeed, private insurance could eventually play a significant role in financing long-term care and could meaningfully reduce out-of-pocket, catastrophic costs and Medicaid expenditures. However, the real-world market penetration is certain to be much less than the simulation because of other barriers to purchase, such as the lack of interest on the part of the nonelderly.

WHY PUBLIC STRATEGIES SHOULD TAKE THE LEAD

Private insurance can and should play a larger role than it does now in financing long-term care. But it is not a panacea. Given the limits of the private sector, greater attention should be given to reforming our public programs.

There are two broad public approaches to financing long-term care. Either we can continue to use the means-tested, welfare program–Medicaid–as the principal government program to finance care, but liberalize it so that it does not require total impoverishment, or we can provide more

FIGURE 1. Private Long-Term Care Insurance Simulation Assumptions

- All persons purchase insurance policies that cover 2 or 4 years of nursing home and home care and pay an initial indemnity value of $60 per day for nursing home care and $30 per visit for home care in 1986. Indemnity values increase by 5.5 percent per year on a compound basis. Premiums for nonelderly increase by 5.5 percent per year until age 65 and then are level. All nondisabled persons who meet affordability criteria buy as much insurance as they can afford.

- *5 PERCENT INCOME*: All elderly purchase policies if they can afford them for 5 percent of their income or less and if they have $10,000 or more in nonhousing assets.

- *MEDICAID INSURANCE:* Elderly who purchase private long-term care insurance may receive Medicaid nursing home benefits while retaining liquid assets beyond what is normally allowed. The additional assets that they keep equal the amount that the private insurance policy pays out in benefits. All elderly purchase policies when they can afford them for 7 percent of their income or less and if they have $10,000 or more in nonhousing assets.

- *TAX FAVORED INSURANCE:* Provides an income-related tax credit of up to 20 percent of the premium cost for elderly purchasing insurance. All elderly purchase policies when they can afford them for 5 percent of their income or less and if they have $10,000 or more in nonhousing assets.

- *EMPLOYER SPONSORED INSURANCE*: Persons as young as age 40 purchase group or individual long-term care insurance policies. Nonelderly purchase policies if premiums are between 2 percent and 4 percent of income (depending on age). Elderly purchase policies if they can afford them for 5 percent or less of income and if they have $10,000 or more in nonhousing assets.

- *ACCELERATED DEATH BENEFITS*: Persons with cash value life insurance use it to finance their nursing home stay. The amount they use is 2.5 percent a month of the life insurance face amount, following a six-month deductible.

long-term care on a nonmeans-tested basis through social insurance. These two approaches need not be mutually exclusive. Indeed, many reform proposals combine the two strategies and include a role for private insurance as well.

A Means-Tested, Medicaid Strategy

Proposals for Medicaid reform generally include using more lenient financial eligibility standards–raising the level of protected assets and

TABLE 2. How Much Can Private Insurance Do? Simulation Results for Four Major Options, 2018

Option	Elderly with Private Insurance[a]	Total Long-Term Care Spending Paid by Private Insurance	Private Insurance Spending on Nursing Home Patients with Incomes > $40,000[c]	Reductions in Medicaid Nursing Home Spending[d]	Reductions in Catastrophic Out-of-Pocket Spending for Nursing Home Patients[e]
Five-percent income	20%	9%	70%	−2%	−6%
Medicaid insurance	32%	14%	61%	−4%	−11%
Tax-favored insurance	28%	12%	64%	−3%	−8%
Employer-sponsored	80%	35%	26%	−32%	−28%
Accelerated death benefits	65%	1%	31%	−1%	0

SOURCE: Brookings-ICF Long-Term Care Financing Model.

[a]Age at initial participation is 67 for all options. Consequently, all are expressed as the percentage of elderly aged 67 and older.
[b]Total long-term care expenditures vary by option.
[c]Income is presented in 1993 dollars.
[d]Medicaid nursing home expenditures for the base case are $49 billion.
[e]Defined as > 40% of income and nonhousing assets.

increasing the amount of income nursing home patients can retain for personal needs–and expanding home care coverage. By liberalizing Medicaid eligibility criteria, the safety net can be cast more widely so that fewer people face complete impoverishment before receiving benefits. In the current political environment, eligibility criteria are likely to be ratcheted down, or tightened, rather than liberalized.

The most compelling argument for means-testing is that it targets public expenditures to those persons with the greatest financial need. In the context of long-term care, advocates of the continued dependence on Medicaid believe that the proper role of government is to finance only that part of care that is beyond the resources of the elderly. People with high levels of income should either purchase private insurance or pay for their care out-of-pocket.

There are, however, several drawbacks to a welfare strategy. Because Medicaid will help fund care only after the disabled have depleted their income and assets, it cannot prevent the elderly from incurring catastrophic costs. Moreover, because benefits are only available to the impoverished, there exists a perverse incentive to transfer, under-report, or shelter wealth of any appreciable size. Perhaps the most disconcerting aspect of using a means-tested program to finance most public long-term care is that it results in a significant number of people who have been financially independent all their lives ending up on welfare. An underlying assumption of welfare programs is that only a relatively small proportion of the population should depend on them. Yet, with long-term care, it is the many, not the few, who rely on welfare in the form of Medicaid.

Nonmeans-Tested Approaches to Long-Term Care

A social insurance approach to financing long-term care offers coverage regardless of financial status. This approach explicitly recognizes long-term care as a normal risk of growing old. Advocates of social insurance see no cogent reason why long-term care should be primarily financed through a welfare program, while acute health care and income support for the elderly are financed through the nonmeans-tested programs of Medicare and Social Security.

Social insurance is the only approach that guarantees universal or near-universal coverage. That is, social insurance covers the able-bodied and the currently disabled, the young and the old, and people of all levels of income and wealth. In this way, social insurance avoids the risk of adverse selection that affects private insurance and the administrative costs of screening out high risks.

Because social insurance programs provide benefits without regard to income, they have the political advantage of including middle- and upper-class beneficiaries as part of their political constituency. These beneficiaries generally wield more political power than the impoverished, and programs benefitting them, such as Social Security and Medicare, tend to be more politically stable than are programs for the poor.

The primary disadvantage of a social insurance approach to financing long-term care is that all proposals would cost the government a significant amount of money. The combination of an intractable budget deficit and resistance to new taxes makes this a formidable barrier. Added to this are the fears of an uncertain national economic future, and the costs associated with a rapidly aging population.

Examination of Four Social Insurance Prototypes

Since 1988, several specific social insurance proposals have been introduced in Congress to cover long-term care. All of these plans provide fairly comprehensive home care. While similar in many ways, these proposals are generally distinguished by the type and duration of nursing home coverage they provide.

Home care-only strategies. Under this design, no major changes would be made to nursing home coverage, but a wide variety of in-home services would be offered. There are several reasons to concentrate on home care. Foremost, the disabled elderly prefer home care because it allows them to maintain a sense of independence, helps reduce unmet care needs, lessens their feelings of being a burden on relatives, and increases their confidence that they will receive the services they need. Home care programs can help caregivers by offering respite from their daily responsibilities.

Improving access to services in the home and thus creating a more balanced delivery system has great appeal. However, nursing home care, not home care, is the major cause of catastrophic costs and welfare dependency among the elderly (Coughlin, Liu, & McBride, 1992). A home care-only strategy would do little to address these problems.

Home care and front-end nursing home coverage. A second strategy would similarly cover comprehensive home care but also provide public insurance for the first part, or "front-end," of a nursing home stay (e.g., the first six months). The rationale for providing front-end coverage is that incremental public expenditures should be concentrated on people who are living in the community or who have the greatest probability of returning home after a nursing home stay. Most persons discharged alive from nursing homes have relatively short lengths of stay (Spence & Wiener, 1990).

Among the limitations of this type of strategy for reform is the fact that many people can already afford to finance short nursing home stays. This approach does little to assist people with long lengths of stay and very large nursing home bills. It is for this reason that this proposal is often combined with liberalization of Medicaid financial eligibility rules.

Home care and back-end nursing home coverage. A third strategy would offer comprehensive home care, but only provide nursing home coverage after a very long deductible period (the so-called "back-end" of a nursing home stay). This approach explicitly assumes that insurers will broadly offer, and large majorities of elderly will purchase, private long-term care insurance to fill in the costly deductible period. Here, in theory at least, private and public insurance are neatly combined into a package where public insurance offers a "backstop" to private coverage.

The strongest argument for back-end coverage is that it would have the government paying for the unquestionably catastrophic costs of long nursing home stays, a role that many feel is most appropriate. However, the reliance on a vast expansion of private-sector insurance makes back-end coverage a high-risk strategy because so few elderly currently have any kind of private coverage.

Another disadvantage to back-end coverage is that few of the long-stay patients targeted by such an approach are discharged alive (Spence & Wiener, 1990). Thus, it provides asset protection for heirs–arguably a less appropriate role for government.

Comprehensive coverage for home care and nursing home care. A fourth strategy, comprehensive coverage, covers comprehensive nursing home and home care after a relatively short deductible period and with moderate coinsurance levels. This strategy seeks to directly solve the problems of long-term care within the structure of a government program, without relying on private insurance to fill the gaps. This approach has the advantage of establishing a single payer, thus enabling the government to control payment rates and how services are delivered. Of all the options, a comprehensive strategy would be best at financing needed care, reducing catastrophic costs, and equalizing access to nursing home care and home care.

The costs of a comprehensive program, however, would be by far the highest of all the social insurance approaches, and other spending priorities would be squeezed. There is also the risk that the system will become rigid and bureaucratic, and unable to respond to the needs of disabled individuals.

Raising the Money

Any responsible new public program for long-term care will need to avoid adding to the federal budget deficit. From a long-term care policy perspective, any number of financing sources would be acceptable so long as enough money were raised to pay for the program. Potential sources include payroll, income, value-added, estate, cigarette, and alcohol taxes; insurance premiums; and Medicare, Medicaid, and other program savings. Politically, of course, raising significant new taxes has stood in the way of public expansion of long-term care and health care for the uninsured, more generally.

Public Program Simulation Results

To evaluate the various types of public long-term care options, Medicaid liberalization and the four social insurance prototypes were simulated. Figure 2 summarizes the simulation assumptions and Tables 3 and 4 summarize the results. All of the social insurance prototypes include changes to the Medicaid program.

Incremental public spending for these options in 1993 for fully implemented programs vary from $6.0 billion for Medicaid liberalization to $49.1 billion for a comprehensive long-term care program. In 2018, these incremental expenditures are projected to vary from $4.3 billion to $109.4 billion for these same options. These expenditures are only for the elderly; including the nonelderly disabled would increase the level of expenditures. Although critics of public insurance approaches argue that incremental expenditures will be largely for the upper-income elderly, the simulations suggest that the overwhelming majority of new spending will be for elderly persons with incomes below $40,000. Finally, compared to the private insurance options, public options do a better job of reducing catastrophic out-of-pocket costs.

Given the fact that all options will require additional public spending, Table 4 offers an illustration of what level of taxation would be required to pay for the various reform options with a payroll tax. Assuming that every dollar of earnings is subject to the payroll tax, a 1.28% payroll tax in 1993 and 3.43% payroll tax in 2048 (employer and employee portions combined) would be required to finance existing public programs on a payroll tax basis (they are not currently financed this way). For the various options, the total public costs would require between a 1.48% and 2.80% payroll tax in 1993. Projected to the year 2048, these rates range from 3.83% to 7.75%. Considering the fact that this payroll tax would be additional to Social Security and Medicare, these are not trivial expenditures,

FIGURE 2. Medicaid Liberalization and Social Insurance Simulation Assumptions

- *MEDICAID LIBERALIZATION:* Medicaid financial eligibility standards increased to allow single individuals and married couples to keep $30,000 and $60,000, respectively, in nonhousing assets. Personal needs allowance increased to $100 per month. Home care for severely disabled expanded and available to persons below 150 percent of federal poverty level. Private insurance available for nursing home and home care.

- *EXPANDED HOME CARE ONLY:* Broad, nonmeans-tested home care coverage of unlimited duration provided to severely disabled elderly (persons with problems with 2 or more activities of daily living [ADLs] or substantial cognitive impairment). Twenty percent coinsurance rate; Medicaid pays coinsurance for population below 150 percent of poverty level. Medicaid liberalization changes listed above included. Private insurance available for nursing home care available.

- *FRONT-END NURSING HOME AND EXPANDED HOME CARE:* Combines Home Care Only program with coverage of first six months of nursing home stay. Twenty percent coinsurance for nursing home care. Medicaid liberalization changes listed above included. Private insurance available for uncovered period of nursing home stays.

- *BACK-END NURSING AND EXPANDED HOME CARE:* Combines Home Care Only program with unlimited nursing home coverage after a two-year deductible period. Twenty percent coinsurance for nursing home care. Medicaid liberalization changes listed above included. Private insurance available to cover two-year deductible period.

- *COMPREHENSIVE NURSING HOME AND EXPANDED HOME CARE:* Combines Home Care Only program with unlimited nursing home coverage with no deductible. Twenty percent coinsurance for nursing home care. Medicaid liberalization changes listed above included. No private insurance available to fill in coinsurance.

but neither are they enormous. To a significant degree, they are expenses that society as a whole will incur, with or without a new program.

CONCLUSIONS

The principal options for long-term care reform are private insurance, Medicaid liberalization, and public long-term care insurance. This article has used the Brookings-ICF Long-Term Care Financing Model to evaluate each of these options in terms of affordability, distribution of benefits, and ability to reduce catastrophic costs.

TABLE 3. Medicaid Liberalization and Social Insurance Strategies, Simulation Results, 2018

Option	Incremental Public Costs (Billions of 1993 Dollars) 1993	2018	Incremental Public Spending on Nursing Home Patients with Incomes > $40,000[a]	Reductions in Catastrophic Out-of-Pocket Spending for Nursing Home Patients[b]
Medicaid liberalization	6.0	4.3	10%	−21%
Social Insurance[c]				
Expanded home care only	20.8	35.2	0%[d]	−23%
Front-end nursing home and expanded home care	23.2	44.5	19%	−31%
Back-end nursing home and expanded care	32.5	66.6	28%	−33%
Comprehensive nursing home and expanded home care	49.1	109.4	26%	−54%

SOURCE: Brookings-ICF Long-Term Care Financing Model.

[a]Income is presented in 1993 dollars.
[b]Defined as > 40% of income and nonhousing assets.
[c]All social insurance strategies include liberalized Medicaid benefits.
[d]Incremental public spending for the elderly with incomes > $40,000 actually decreased under this option because of the purchase of private insurance among this group.

The simulation results for private long-term care insurance suggest that the industry is at a crossroads. So long as private insurance is aimed principally at the elderly population, its market penetration and ability to finance long-term care will remain severely limited, even substantially into the future. Because of limited market penetration, private insurance will not substantially reduce the level of catastrophic costs among the elderly. Moreover, private insurance expenditures will be made mostly on behalf of the upper-income elderly. As a result, private insurance sold to the elderly will have almost no impact on Medicaid expenditures.

The situation would change substantially if companies could be convinced to offer private long-term care insurance to their active employees and if workers were willing to buy the product. The simulation results clearly suggest that the affordability problem can largely be solved by

TABLE 4. Total Expenditures for Public Long-Term Care as a Percentage of Payroll for the Base-Case and Public Insurance Options, Selected Periods (Billions of 1993 Dollars)

	Payroll Tax[a]		
Option	1993	2018	2048[b]
Base case			
Total costs	2.37	3.61	6.85
Public costs	1.28	1.80	3.43
Medicaid liberalization	1.48	1.93	3.83
Expanded home care only	1.89	2.42	4.58
Front-end nursing home and expanded home care	1.99	2.59	4.91
Back-end nursing home and expanded care	2.28	3.15	6.08
Comprehensive nursing home and expanded home care	2.80	3.98	7.75

SOURCE: Brookings-ICF Long-Term Care Financing Model.

[a]Combined employee and employer contributions. No ceiling on taxable salaries.
[b]2048 represents the five-year average for the period 2045-2050.

selling properly structured policies to the nonelderly. However, selling policies to the nonelderly in large numbers will be extremely difficult and is likely to take a very long time. Moreover, the financial risks to insurers of selling to the nonelderly are very large.

Since private long-term care insurance is not likely to change the way in which long-term care is financed, greater attention should be paid to reforming public programs. On balance, Medicaid liberalization offers lower incremental cost and concentrates expenditures on the lower-income population. However, there is little public support for means-tested programs and those who do rely on Medicaid often face access problems and services of uncertain quality.

On the other hand, social insurance offers protection for individuals against impoverishment and has the ability to spread the risk of needing long-term care across everyone. But all social insurance strategies are more expensive than Medicaid liberalization. Not surprisingly, the comprehensive option, which does far better than either front-end or back-end options in reducing catastrophic costs (which in turn do better than the private insurance options), is very expensive in terms of public spending.

REFERENCES

American Council on Life Insurance. (1993). *1992 Life insurance fact book update*. Washington, DC: Author.

Coronel, S., & Fulton, D. (1995). *Long-term care insurance in 1993*. Washington, DC: Health Insurance Association of America.

Coughlin, T. A., Liu, K., & McBride, T. D. (1992). Severely disabled elderly persons with financially catastrophic health care expenses: Sources and determinants. *The Gerontologist*, *32*, 391-403.

Crown, W. H., Capitman, J., & Leutz, W. L. (1992). Economic rationality, the affordability of private long-term care insurance, and the role for public policy. *The Gerontologist*, *32*, 478-485.

Friedland, R. (1990). *Facing the costs of long-term care: An EBRI-ERF policy study*. Washington, DC: Employee Benefit Research Institute.

LifePlans. (1992). *Who buys long-term care insurance*? Washington, DC: Health Insurance Association of America.

Manton, D. G., Corder, L. S., & Stallard, E. (1993). Estimates of change in chronic disability and institutional incidence and prevalence rates in the U.S. elderly population from the 1982, 1984, and 1989 National Long Term Care Survey. *Journal of Gerontology: Social Science*, *48*, S153-166.

Rivlin, A. M., Wiener, J. M., Spence, D. A., & Hanley, R. J. (1988). *Caring for the disabled elderly: Who will pay*? Washington, DC: The Brookings Institution.

Spence, D. A., & Wiener, J. M. (1990). Nursing home length of stay patterns: Results from the 1985 National Nursing Home Survey. *The Gerontologist*, *30*, 16-20.

Wiener, J. M., Illston, L. H., & Hanley, R. J. (1994). *Sharing the burden: strategies for public and private long-term care insurance*. Washington, DC: The Brookings Institution.

Zedlewski, S. R., Barnes, R. A., Burt, M. A., McBride, T. D., & Meyer, J. (1990). *The needs of the elderly in the 21st century*. Washington, DC: Urban Institute Press.

Designing Home Care Benefits: The Range of Options and Experience

Vicki A. Freedman, PhD

RAND
Washington, DC

Peter Kemper, PhD

Center for Studying Health System Change
Washington, DC

Vicki Freedman is a population epidemiologist with RAND in Washington, DC. She was formerly with the Agency for Health Care Policy and Research. Peter Kemper is Deputy Director of the Center for Studying Health System Change. His research focuses on managed care and long-term care.

The authors wish to thank Diane Justice, Patrick Hennessy, Ann Barr, Lisa Alecxih, and many others consulted for providing valuable information on current practice; Bob Applebaum, Ann Barr, Marc Cohen, Diane Justice, Katie Maslow, Jim Reschovsky, Bill Spector, and Joshua Wiener for helpful comments on an earlier version of the paper; Dawn French for secretarial support; and Sheri Gerstein for providing invaluable research assistance for the project as a Somers intern through the National Academy for Social Insurance.

The views expressed in the paper are those of the authors. No official endorsement by either the Department of Health and Human Services or the Agency for Health Care Policy and Research is intended or should be inferred.

Vicki Freedman can be contacted care of RAND, 2100 M Street, NW, Washington, DC 20037.

[Haworth co-indexing entry note]: "Designing Home Care Benefits: The Range of Options and Experience." Freedman, Vicki A. and Peter Kemper. Co-published simultaneously in *Journal of Aging & Social Policy* (The Haworth Press, Inc.) Vol. 7, No. 3/4, 1996, pp. 129-148; and: *From Nursing Homes to Home Care* (ed: Marie E. Cowart and Jill Quadagno) The Haworth Press, Inc., 1996, pp. 129-148. Single or multiple copies of this article are available from The Haworth Document Delivery Service [1-800-342-9678, 9:00 a.m. - 5:00 p.m. (EST)].

SUMMARY. This article presents a framework identifying important home care benefit design decisions and reviews existing designs that have been adopted in practice. Four basic designs were identified, based on a review of 55 home care benefits drawn from public programs in the United States and foreign countries, and from private long-term care insurance policies in the United States. Three of these designs–service entitlements, managed-service benefits, and cash disability allowances–have each been adopted by public programs in the United States and abroad, and by private insurance policies in the United States. A fourth design–individualized cash benefits–has been adopted in only one experimental program. The designs observed in practice are remarkably varied, providing evidence that many alternative designs are feasible. Experimentation, particularly with cash disability allowances, is needed to determine the relative costs and benefits of various designs. *[Article copies available from The Haworth Document Delivery Service: 1-800-342-9678.]*

Over the past decade, public funding of home care services in the United States has been increasing. States have been expanding public home care programs for low-income groups through a combination of general revenue programs, Medicaid waivers, and federal block grants. As more public home care programs are initiated or expanded, how best to design such programs becomes an increasingly important issue for policymakers. Despite its relevance, the design of home and community-based service programs has been the subject of few systematic analyses. This article addresses one aspect of home care design, the design of the benefit–what it is, and who controls its use and provision. Specifically, the article has two goals: (1) to develop a framework that identifies the important benefit design decisions and (2) to identify the range of designs that have been adopted and characterize common practice.

FRAMEWORK

A great many issues must be considered in designing a home care program–what benefits will be covered, how the program is financed, who is eligible–to name a few. The focus in this article is on benefit design issues that have the greatest effect on the allocation of covered services among an eligible population and, therefore, are likely to have the greatest effect on cost and quality-of-life outcomes. The discussion here is restricted to a benefit providing home and community-based care to older persons with severe disabilities, with *personal* care being the dominant service. Three benefit design issues were identified that are likely to affect the cost and outcomes of a program (see Table 1).

The first and most important issue is the type of benefit. Two fundamental questions determine the "basic benefit type." The first is whether the benefit is restricted to services or is a cash payment that can be spent without restriction. This distinction is not simply a matter of whether beneficiaries receive cash or services. If beneficiaries receive cash payments but are required to submit receipts for services or have checks

TABLE 1. Fundamental Home Care Benefit Design Questions

Basic Benefit Type

What type of benefits are provided?

- Services
- Cash that can be spent without restrictions

How is the benefit level determined?

- Individual and/or provider decides (subject to program rules)
- Agent of the payer decides on case-by-case basis

Covered Services and Providers

What services are covered?

- Only a single service or few services
- A defined list of a wide range of home care services
- Any approved service needed to meet home care needs

Who can provide covered services?

- Approved agencies
- Individual providers
- Family members

Control Over Service Mix and Provider

Who has the authority over the mix of services used?

- The client (with advice of provider or case manager)
- An agent of the payer (in consultation with the client)

Who chooses the provider?

- The client (with advice of a case manager or physician)
- An agent of the payer (in consultation with the client)

co-signed by providers, then the benefit is effectively restricted to services. The second question is how the level of benefits is determined. The level may be determined by the home care client or the provider, subject to program rules. Alternatively, an agent of the payer, such as a case manager, may determine the amount of benefits on a case-by-case basis, given information about the beneficiary's needs and resources.

The answers to these two questions define the four basic benefit types shown in Table 2. A *service entitlement* covers services to which beneficiaries are entitled according to rules defined by law, in program regulations, or in a contract. The amount of the benefit is determined by the beneficiary or provider subject to these rules and typically an ex-post review or audit of expenditures to ensure compliance. Like service entitlements, *managed-service benefits* are also limited to services; however, an agent of the payer determines the amount of the benefit. Typically, professional judgment determines the level of each individual's benefit, although guidelines are sometimes used to ensure that similarly situated clients are treated equally. The third type of benefit, a *disability allowance,* pays cash to persons who satisfy well-defined eligibility rules without restricting what can be purchased. The amount of the cash payment may vary according to specified rules, for example, based on the level of disability. Finally, an *individualized cash benefit* is a cash payment without restriction as to use but in an amount that is determined by an agent of the payer based on a judgment about the individual's needs and circumstances.

Given a basic benefit design, two additional sets of design decisions concern (1) the range of covered services and providers and (2) control over the mix of services and the choice of providers. For disability allowances and individualized cash benefits, these decisions are implicit in the basic benefit designs: by definition, the beneficiary is free to determine which goods and

TABLE 2. Basic Home Care Benefit Designs

	Benefits Restricted to Services?	
Does an Agent of Payer Determine the Benefit Level?	Services only	Unrestricted cash
No	Service Entitlement[a]	Disability Allowance[b]
Yes	Managed Service Benefit	Individualized Cash Benefits

[a]Individual or provider decides benefit level within benefit rules and subject to ex-post review of benefits paid.
[b]Benefit level determined by pre-existing program rules.

services to purchase and from whom. These decisions are important design issues, however, for both service entitlements and managed-service benefits.

In developing the framework and presenting examples of benefit designs, there has been an attempt to make clear distinctions among the design options. These distinctions are not always clear-cut in practice; as a consequence, the characterization of specific programs here may in some instances be open to debate. Nevertheless, emphasizing the polar distinctions among design choices allows clarification of the available alternatives in designing home care benefits.

SOURCES OF INFORMATION

Using the framework described above, the experience of 55 home care programs was reviewed. To identify the broadest possible range of designs, examples were drawn from public programs in the United States and foreign countries, and from private long-term care insurance policies in the United States. The selection of specific benefit designs to be reviewed for this project was driven by a number of considerations. First, the relatively limited extent of written materials was a constraint; this was particularly true regarding foreign programs. A variety of sources were therefore used, including published literature, unpublished reports, program documents, insurance contracts, and interviews with experts in the field. A second consideration was the aim of the study to identify as wide a range of designs as possible. Thus, a number of designs were chosen purposefully to represent a unique home care benefit design feature. This is particularly true regarding the selection of private insurance policies. Finally, there was a desire to cover the experience of relatively well-funded state home care programs. States rely on three major sources of funding for home and community-based services: Medicaid waivers, Medicaid's optional personal care benefit, and state general revenue programs. To the extent possible, Medicaid optional personal care benefit programs and state general revenue programs with the highest per capita expenditures were chosen for review. In addition, because Donna Folkemer (1994) and Diane Justice (1993) have recently surveyed Medicaid waiver programs in detail, their reports were relied on for waiver program information.

The 55 designs reviewed included three federally administered programs, 17 state general revenue programs, 8 Medicaid optional personal care benefit programs, 17 programs in 9 foreign countries, and 10 private insurance policies from 7 companies. A list of designs reviewed is provided in Table 3. A report describing these home and community-based programs in detail (Gerstein, 1994) is available from the authors.

TABLE 3. Designs Reviewed

FEDERAL PROGAMS
- State Supplemental Payments to the Supplemental Security Income
- Medicare Home Health
- VA Housebound and Aid & Attendance Allowance

STATE PROGRAMS

State General Revenue
- California In-Home Supportive Services
- Colorado Home Care Allowance
- Connecticut Home Care Program for Elders
- Iowa In-Home Health-Related Care Services
- Indiana CHOICE
- Illinois Community Care
- Maine Home Based Care
- Maine Self-Directed Voucher Demonstration
- Massachusetts Home Care
- Michigan Care Management
- North Dakota SPED
- New York EISEP
- Oklahoma Home Maintenance Aid Services
- Oregon Project Independence
- Rhode Island CORE
- Rhode Island Copay
- Wisconsin Community Options Program

Medicaid Personal Care
- Arkansas
- District of Columbia
- Maryland
- Michigan
- Montana
- New York
- Oklahoma
- Texas

INTERNATIONAL PROGRAMS
- Australia
- Austria
- British Columbia, Canada
- Germany
- Israel
- Manitoba, Canada
- Netherlands
- Sweden
- United Kingdom

PRIVATE INSURANCE POLICIES
- Aetna Employer-Sponsored Long-Term Care Insurance
- Bankers Life & Casualty Long-Term Care Insurance
- Blue Cross & Blue Shield of Connecticut Generations
- CNA Preferred Advantage
- John Hancock Protectcare
- TIAA Long Term Care Insurance
- UNUM Advantage I and Advantage II

Because information was available for some programs or insurance policies but not others, the designs reviewed do not necessarily constitute a representative sample. Although the information available satisfies the objective of providing examples of the range of designs, generalization is sometimes difficult. Where a pattern appears strong, however, generalizations are ventured here–with the recognition that caution is necessary.

FINDINGS

Basic Benefit Type

Three basic benefit designs–service entitlements, managed-service benefits, and cash disability allowances–have all been adopted in the United States, abroad, and by private insurers; only one program has adopted an individualized cash benefit design (see Table 4). In general, coverage of services is far more common than unrestricted cash payments.

Service entitlement. A good example of a service entitlement in the United States is Medicare's home health benefit. Medicare pays for services in the home for beneficiaries who are (1) homebound, (2) under a plan of care established by a physician, and (3) require the use of one or more qualifying skilled services. Covered services include skilled nursing, home health aide visits, medical social services, and physical speech and occupational therapies. Although a physician is technically required to certify medical necessity, decisions about services are, in practice, made by the home health provider within the Medicare rules. Fiscal intermediaries review claims after they are paid to determine compliance.

States generally have not adopted service entitlement designs for their home care programs. Two exceptions are personal care benefits under the Medicaid program in Arkansas and Montana, both of which are service entitlements. These programs mirror Medicare's home health benefit in that the provider (typically a nurse of the provider agency) determines the benefit level within Medicaid rules. Service entitlements are also uncommon in the foreign countries we reviewed. The only examples found were relatively small programs in Germany and Austria that were part of systems with much larger disability allowances (these are discussed later).

In contrast with public programs, service entitlements (or "incurred expense indemnities") are the dominant design for private insurance policies (personal communication, Lisa Alecxih).[1] This may be because the private insurance market, which is relatively young, grew out of the fee-for-service health insurance market where indemnity policies have been

TABLE 4. Examples of Basic Home Care Benefit Designs

Basic Benefit Type	United States	International	Private Insurance
Service entitlement	Medicare Home Health	Austria (service program)	CNA Basic Benefit
	Medicaid Personal Care Benefit	Germany (service option)	Bankers Life
	Arkansas		John Hancock Basic Benefit
	Montana		TIAA
Managed service benefit	17/17 State general revenue	Australia HACC	Blue Cross of Connecticut
	42/42 Medicaid Waiver[a]	Australia COPS	CNA Alternative Care Plan
	Medicaid Personal Care	British Columbia	John Hancock Alternate Care Plan
	District of Columbia	Israel	
	Maryland	Manitoba	
	Michigan	Netherlands	
	New York	Netherlands experiment (service option)	
	Oklahoma	Sweden	
	Texas	United Kingdom	
Disability allowance	Veteran's Attendance Allowance	Austria (cash program)	UNUM
	SSI State Supplements	Germany (cash option)	Aetna
Individualized cash benefit		Netherlands experiment (cash option)	

[a]Justice (1992)

the norm. Such policies typically cover expenses for a specified list of services up to a daily maximum; once a policyholder fulfills disability requirements specified in the insurance contract, he or she is entitled to home care services under the policy's rules subject to any policy limits and to the insurer's review of claims submitted.

Managed-service benefits. The managed-service benefit is the dominant design among public programs in the United States. All 17 of the state general-revenue programs reviewed for this study and all 42 Medicaid waiver programs serving the aged and disabled surveyed by Justice (1993) are managed-service benefits. The Medicaid optional personal-care benefit also has been implemented as a managed-service benefit in a number of states with relatively large programs where state case-workers or state-employed nurses determine the benefit amount.

The managed-service benefit was also the dominant design in the foreign programs reviewed in this study. The Canadian provinces of British Columbia and Manitoba, along with Australia, Israel, the Netherlands, Sweden, and the United Kingdom, have all adopted home and community-based care designs under which eligible applicants may receive a benefit in-kind. Benefits are restricted to services and, with the exception of Israel, the level of the benefit is determined on a case-by-case basis by a representative of the program (personal communication, Patrick Hennessy, 1994). In Israel, a nurse who is an agent of the state determines the amount of services an individual receives based on rules that translate disability into benefit level. This system was designed with the intended goal of providing the same benefit level to similarly situated individuals (Factor, Morgenstin, & Naon, 1992).

Private insurers are beginning to develop policies that rely on case managers to determine the level of benefits. For example, Blue Cross of Connecticut offers a policy that covers a broad range of services managed by a case manager. When a policyholder meets the policy's disability criteria, a "personal care advocate" develops a care plan to make efficient use of the policy's benefits, which are subject to a dollar limit over the lifetime of the policyholder. In addition, some incurred expense indemnity policies, such as those offered by CNA and John Hancock, have "alternate care provisions," which are managed-service benefits. Under these provisions, the insured is offered the option of using benefits at a level below the daily maximum in order to stretch the policy's maximum lifetime benefit over a longer period of time. Such alternate care plans must be approved by the insurer's case manager.

Disability allowance. Among public programs, disability allowances typically are not recognized as long-term care benefits because they are part of social welfare or pension programs. In some cases, care coordination services may be offered in conjunction with cash disability allowances, but the information is only advisory; the ultimate choice of how to spend the allowance is left to the consumer.

The Housebound and Aid and Attendance Allowance Program of the Department of Veterans' Affairs exemplifies the disability allowance approach. Since 1951, the Department has provided allowances to disabled veterans with service-related disabilities and to low-income veterans with nonservice-related disabilities. The cash benefit, which varies according to disability level, is added to the beneficiary's pension check and may be spent in any manner the veteran chooses (Grana & Yamashiro, 1987).

An example of disability allowances that are part of a welfare rather than a pension program are certain State Supplemental Payments under the federal Supplemental Security Income (SSI) program. SSI provides income support payments to elderly, blind, and disabled persons meeting income and asset requirements. States are permitted to make additional payments to individuals qualifying for SSI. Nineteen states make additional cash payments to older persons with special health-related needs with the express intention of allowing recipients to remain in their homes. One state makes Supplemental Payments to persons living independently and receiving SSI because of disability rather than age (Neuschler, 1987). Such payments are made without requirements that recipients purchase services.[2]

Other countries have also adopted the disability allowance approach. In 1988, Germany added a limited home care benefit to its health insurance benefit package. Individuals who meet disability requirements can receive home care benefits in the form of services up to a maximum number of visits or as an unrestricted cash payment of fixed value (set at about half the cost of the maximum number of visits).[3] Under recently passed legislation, this disability payment will be expanded substantially, and the amount of the cash payment will vary based on the level of the individual's disability (Alber, 1992). Austria also has recently reformed its cash attendance allowance, or *Pflegegeld.* Since 1993, the allowance has been awarded at one of seven different rates that vary according to the degree of need (Hörl, 1993). Unlike the German program, which offers a choice between services and a cash benefit, the Austrian allowance program offers only a cash benefit.[4]

Finally, at least two private insurers have adopted disability allowances. Aetna and UNUM both offer policies that pay a fixed daily amount of cash to persons who become disabled.

Individualized cash benefit. In this review, only one program was encountered that has adopted an individualized cash benefit. From 1991 to 1993, the Dutch government financed a small experiment to study cash benefits as an alternative to in-kind services. The amount of cash offered to participants who were randomized to an experimental group was based upon an individualized care plan developed by a social worker in consultation with the client (Cameron & Firman, 1995).

Other than the Dutch experiment, this study did not find any other public program in the United States or abroad or any insurance policy that bases the amount of a cash benefit on case-by-case judgments about individual need. A number of state programs–such as the Colorado Home Care Allowance and the Wisconsin Community Options Program–permit varying cash payments to eligible applicants; these programs have been classified elsewhere as "cash and counseling" (Cameron & Firman, 1995). In the framework of this study, however, these benefits are managed-service benefits because the disbursements are restricted to the purchase of services (broadly defined).

Covered Services

As shown in Table 5, existing service entitlements and managed-service benefits offer a variety of home and community-based services to older frail persons.

Service entitlements. The public service entitlements reviewed cover only a single or very limited set of services. Although clarifications to the Medicare rules in 1989 regarding service coverage have increased the number of (unskilled) home health aide visits, Medicare's home health benefit was initially (and is still largely) limited to skilled, medically oriented home health care, skilled nursing care, therapies, or assistance from a medical social worker. Similarly, as indicated, the Medicaid optional personal care benefit limits service coverage to a single service–assistance with personal care activities such as bathing, dressing and eating.[5] The service entitlements identified abroad also limit the array of services covered. The in-kind component of the German long-term care program limits benefits to nursing visits. Austria's in-kind services are limited to nursing and personal care.

In contrast with public programs, private insurance policies that are service entitlements cover a broader–but still defined–list of services. All four service indemnity plans reviewed for this analysis cover home help, personal care, skilled nursing, adult day care, and respite services.

Managed-service benefits. In the United States, managed-service benefits most commonly cover a broad range of services, with coverage of a

TABLE 5. Covered Services

	United States	Foreign	Private Insurance
Service Entitlement			
Single or very limited	Medicare Home Health Medicaid Personal Care Arkansas Montana	Austria (service component) Germany (service component)	--
Defined list	--	--	Bankers Life CNA Basic Benefit John Hancock Basic Benefit TIAA
Full Range[a]	--	--	--
Managed Service Benefit			
Single or very limited	4/17 State general revenue 4/43 Medicaid waiver[b] Medicaid Personal Care District of Columbia Maryland Michigan New York Oklahoma Texas	--	--
Defined list	11/17 State general revenue 38/43 Medicaid waiver[b]	Australia HACC British Columbia Israel Manitoba Sweden Netherlands United Kingdom	Blue Cross of Connecticut John Hancock Alternate Care Plan
Full range[a]	2/17 State general revenue 1/43 Medicaid waiver[b]	Australia COPS	CNA Alternate Care Plan

[a]Covers any service intended to meet the client's long-term care needs at home.
[b]Folkemer (1993)

defined list of services most common. Most Medicaid waiver programs cover a standard package of benefits including home help, personal care, skilled nursing and therapy services, adult day care, transportation, and so forth (Folkemer, 1994). Among the state general revenue programs reviewed in this study, the majority cover a defined list of services. In contrast, managed-service benefits funded under the Medicaid personal care option cover a very limited range of services, reflecting the nature of the benefit as defined by federal rules.

Other countries providing managed-service benefits also commonly cover a defined list of services. For example, although designs vary across localities, the Netherlands, Sweden and the United Kingdom cover home help, personal care services, and skilled nursing services (Monk & Cox, 1991). Australia's Home and Community Care Program (Howe, 1992) and Manitoba's Home Care Program (Monk & Cox, 1989) cover not only home help, personal care, and skilled nursing but also respite care, meals-on-wheels, home modifications, transportation, and medical supplies.

As indicated, relatively few private insurers offer managed-service benefit policies. Two of the three policies reviewed in this study covered a defined list of services, and the third, CNA's alternate plan of care benefit, permits payments for anything that will help the policyholder to stay at home, by agreement among the insured party, his or her physician, and CNA.

Covered Providers

A continuum of options exists with respect to the providers covered (see Table 6): contracting with a single organization to provide all services; using a list of agencies meeting program requirements, either through contractual arrangement or a certification process; allowing beneficiaries to contract directly with individual providers; and permitting payments to family members.

Service entitlements. The public service entitlements encompass a variety of approaches to defining allowable service providers. At one extreme, the state of Montana's optional personal care benefit provides services through a single agency.[6] Somewhat less restrictive is the Medicare home health benefit, which pays providers affiliated with any home health agency certified by the program. Both Germany's and Austria's service components require providers to be affiliated with an agency. No public service entitlements identified in this study allowed payments to individual providers or family members.

Private-service indemnity policies also vary with respect to covered providers. Bankers Life and John Hancock insurance companies allow

TABLE 6. Allowed Providers

	United States	Foreign	Private Insurance
Service Entitlement			
Approved agencies only	Medicare Home Health Medicaid Personal Care Arkansas Montana	Austria (service component) Germany (service component)	Bankers Life John Hancock Basic Benefit
Agencies and individuals	--	--	John Hancock Enriched Home Care TIAA
Any provider[a]	--	--	CNA Basic Benefit
Managed Service Benefit			
Approved agencies only	9/17 State general revenue 25/43 Medicaid waiver[c] Medicaid Personal Care New York Texas	Australia COPS Australia HACC British Columbia Israel Manitoba Sweden Netherlands United Kingdom	Blue Cross of Connecticut John Hancock Alternate Care Plan
Agencies and individuals[a]	3/17 State general revenue 8/43 Medicaid waiver[c] Medicaid Personal Care District of Columbia Maryland Oklahoma	--	--
Any provider[b]	5/17 State general revenue 10/43 Medicaid waiver[c] Medicaid Personal Care Michigan	--	CNA Alternate Care Plan

[a]Excludes family providers.
[b]Covers any provider including family, as well as agencies and individuals.
[c] Folkemer (1993).

only approved agencies to provide services; TIAA and John Hancock allow both agency and individual providers but exclude payments to family members; and CNA has no restrictions on who may be paid to provide home care.

Managed-service benefits. Like service entitlements, public programs with managed service benefits in the United States vary with respect to the range of permissible providers. The most common design limits payment to approved agencies. About half the state general revenue programs reviewed for this study and more than half the Medicaid waiver programs for the elderly require agencies to furnish services. Managed-service benefits in foreign countries require participants to use providers affiliated with either governmental or private agencies. The Canadian province of Manitoba, for example, relies on a government-owned delivery system, while the Netherlands provides home care through two voluntary associations, one providing home help and the other providing home nursing (Monk & Cox, 1989). Finally, among private insurers, Blue Cross requires that services be provided through a licensed agency and that hands-on care be provided by a licensed health care professional. John Hancock (under its alternate care plan benefit) restricts providers to licensed home health agencies.[7]

Although restricting providers to approved agencies is most common, an important minority of managed-service benefits in the United States permit provision directly by individual providers. About half the general revenue programs reviewed for this study and just under half the Medicaid waiver programs for the elderly allow the use of individually contracted providers (Folkemer, 1994). Such programs often give participants responsibilities for managing their own provider, including recruiting, hiring, firing, and training. In some cases–for example, in some counties in California–individuals are given a choice between agency and individual providers.

Many of these programs also permit payment to family members. About a third of the general revenue programs reviewed for this study allow payments to family members. Although Medicaid prohibits payment to family members, states have been able to minimize the impact of this requirement by defining "family" narrowly (e.g., spouse or parent of an adult child). As a result, nearly a fourth of all Medicaid waiver programs allow payments to family members under certain circumstances (Folkemer, 1994). In addition, under Michigan's Medicaid personal care benefit, family members provide care to nearly half of all participants (Linsk, Keigher, Simon-Rusinowitz, & England, 1992). Finally, among private insurance, CNA's alternate care plan benefit explicitly permits payment to family members.

Control of Service Mix

For benefits that cover more than a single service, a range of options exists with respect to the control over service mix. At one end, consumers are given full control and responsibility for selecting appropriate services, without the formal participation of an agent of the payer (although the beneficiary may seek advice from providers, family, or a professional care coordinator). At the other extreme, a case manager who is an agent of the payer devises a care plan in consultation with the client and family and authorizes payment for services under this plan.

Very little variation in the control over service mix for either service entitlements or managed service benefits was observed in this study. Although determination of the overall amount of benefits in principle could be separated from determination of the mix of services within that amount, in virtually all the examples studied, the two are determined as part of the same process.

Service entitlements. Among service entitlements reviewed in this study, the provider (in consultation with the beneficiary) develops a plan that determines the level and mix of services simultaneously. No case manager responsible directly to the payer is involved in the care planning. This is true of all the public and private service entitlements for which information was available.

Managed-service benefits. Under managed-service benefits, the level and mix of services are typically determined as part of the same care planning process that determines the level of benefits. Thus, public managed-service benefits in the United States almost always involve an agent of the payer in the authorization of the care plan. Even programs involving cash and referred to as "client-directed"–such as Colorado's Home Care Allowance program and Wisconsin's Community Options Program–involve a case manager and do not leave the care plan determination solely to the client. Similarly, in all the managed-service benefits in foreign countries and in private insurance policies reviewed, an agent of the payer retains ultimate control over the choice of services.

It is not necessary to give authority over both the level and mix of services to an agent of the payer, although it is an almost universal practice to do so in managed-service benefits. A case manager could determine the level of benefits but leave control of the mix of services to the beneficiary, for example, through the use of vouchers. No existing managed-service benefits were encountered that allowed the client the choice of a range of services through vouchers, although two demonstrations that use vouchers were identified in this study.[8]

Choice of provider. Responsibility for choosing a provider can be given to the client, with the advice of family members, providers, or case managers; or to an agent of the payer, in consultation with the client. Between these extreme alternatives, however, there is a range of shared responsibility between the client and the agent of the payer, making characterization of the responsibility difficult in practice.

As with choice of service mix, the extent of choice of provider may be constrained by the range of options permitted. Benefits that cover services from only a single agency by definition restrict the choice to that provider. At the other extreme, designs that permit payment to individually contracted providers typically do so under the assumption that the client will ultimately choose (and in some cases recruit, hire, and potentially fire) the provider.

Service entitlements. All of the service entitlements in U.S. public programs and private insurance, as well as the in-kind option of the German program, leave the choice of providers to the beneficiary. Indeed, Medicaid requires that beneficiaries be given a choice of provider.

Managed service benefits. The Medicaid choice of provider requirement also affects the design of managed-service benefits in the United States. All of the waiver programs surveyed by Justice (1993) and all of the Medicaid personal care programs reviewed here offered clients a choice of providers, as did all but two of the general revenue programs reviewed. Case managers were involved in this choice, however, and information about the extent to which client preferences drive the care planning process was not readily available. Private insurers that offer managed-service benefits also allow the policyholder to select the provider. In contrast, in managed-service benefits abroad, it appears that program agents typically choose the provider, although definitive information was not available.

DISCUSSION

This article has identified three sets of decisions concerning the design of a home and community-based service benefit package: the basic benefit type, coverage of services and providers, and choice of service mix and providers. Depending on these decisions, a great many specific designs are logically possible. While several designs predominate, this review of U.S. and foreign government programs and private long-term care insurance policies identified examples of a wide variety of designs being used in practice.

The wide range of home care benefit designs observed in practice indicates that many alternative designs are feasible and could be adopted by policymakers. The choice among the alternative feasible designs should depend on the specific goals. There are many possible, often conflicting, policy goals for a home care program, including improved quality of life of persons with disability or their family caregivers, efficient use and delivery of services, equitable allocation of services, responsiveness to individual needs, and control of public spending, to name a few. Yet, there is virtually no evidence concerning how alternative designs affect costs and outcomes. Moreover, theoretical analysis provides little guidance about the likely direction or strength of these effects. Consequently, there is currently almost no basis for choosing among the many feasible home care designs.

The lack of evidence suggests the need for experimentation with alternative designs to ensure that public home care budgets are spent in a manner consistent with policy goals. Rigorous evaluations are needed to assess the effects of the alternative designs on costs and quality of life. In most cases, a randomized experimental design would be required. In the absence of such evaluations, the uncertainty about policy-related outcomes is likely to remain even after a demonstration has taken place.

One priority area for experimentation concerns the basic benefit design. As indicated, there is relatively little experience in the United States with disability allowances and none with individualized cash benefits. Cash benefits are inherently controversial because of the uncertainty of their effects. Some argue that costs will be high due to high participation rates, and that quality of care will be poor because of the lack of government control over service provision; others argue that the flexibility afforded by disability allowances will enhance quality of life in the long run. By randomizing program participants to either a fixed cash payment or managed-service benefit, an allowance similar to that of Austria could be evaluated. Alternatively, by randomizing program participants to the choice of either a cash or service benefit, one could test the impact of introducing a hybrid program with either a fixed cash benefit (as in Germany) or an individualized cash benefit (as in the Dutch experiment).

In summary, the home care benefit designs observed in practice are remarkably varied, providing a good deal of experience and a wide range of designs. Information is lacking, however, that ties the various designs to specific policy goals. Investments in our understanding of the effects of alternative home care designs are needed to ensure that public funding is spent on home care designs that best meet policy goals.

ENDNOTES

1. Although incurred-expense indemnity policies dominate the market, their disproportionate share is not reflected here because we purposefully selected a range of designs.

2. Also common are payments to persons living in domiciliary care homes. Currently, 34 states provide payments to disabled persons with special living arrangements. Because these payments require the purchase of a particular service (e.g., domiciliary care), these benefits are service entitlements in our framework rather than disability allowances.

3. The in-kind service option under this hybrid program is a service entitlement. Cameron and Firman (1995) report that the vast majority of recipients choose the cash option.

4. Austria also has a separate in-kind service program that provides nursing and personal care services. The in-kind program is about one tenth the size of the cash allowance program (OECD, 1992).

5. Some of these programs allow providers to perform oversight, emergency assistance, or some paramedical services, but the majority are limited to assistance with personal care.

6. Although in theory this agency encourages program participants to recruit individuals for the agency to hire, in practice, program participants rarely pursue this option and therefore have only available agency staff from which to choose (Kennedy & Litvak, 1991).

7. Under an enriched benefit option that covers homemaker services, however, individual providers may be employed.

8. Maine's Self-Directed Voucher Program, a tiny demonstration incorporated into Maine's existing home care program, allows clients using vouchers to select a personal care provider. The case manager suggests services but does not formally develop a care plan; the client decides the specific types of help to be provided by the personal care attendant. In addition, the Health Care Financing Administration has recently funded an evaluation of a Medicare Voucher Demonstration in New York and West Virginia. The study will randomize over 1,000 home care clients with severe or moderate impairment and a high risk of hospitalization to one of four groups: voucher, nurse case management, voucher and nurse case management, or a control group. Clients randomized to receive vouchers will be able to choose from a broad list of services.

REFERENCES

Alber, J. (1992). *The debate over long-term care insurance in Germany.* University of Konstanz. Prepared for the Organization for Economic Cooperation and Development for the 1992 Meeting on The Care of Frail Elderly People, Paris, November 2-4, 1992.

Cameron, K., & Firman, J.P. (1995). *International and domestic programs using "cash and counseling" strategies to pay for long-term care.* National Council on the Aging.

Connecticut Department of Social Services. (1993). *Procedures and guidelines for self-directed care: Connecticut Home Care Program for Elders*.

Factor, H., Morgenstin, B., & Naon, D. (1992). *Home-care services in Israel*. Joint Israel Brookdale Institute of Gerontology and Adult Human Development.

Folkemer, D. (1994). *State use of home & community-based services for the aged under Medicaid: Waiver programs, personal care, frail elderly services and home health services*. The Intergovernmental Health Policy Project.

Gerstein, S. (1994). *A review of home and community-based care programs: United States, international and private insurance experience*. Prepared for the Agency for Health Care Policy and Research.

Grana, J., & Yamashiro, S. (1987). *An evaluation of the Veterans Administration Housebound and Aid and Attendance Allowance program*. Project Hope report prepared for Office of the Assistant Secretary for Planning and Evaluation.

Hörl, J. (1993). Eldercare policy between the state and family: Austria. *Journal of Aging & Social Policy, 5*, 155-168.

Howe, A. (1992). *The care of the frail elderly: National report, Australia*. Prepared for the Organization for Economic Cooperation and Development for the 1992 Meeting on The Care of Frail Elderly People, Paris, November 2-4, 1992.

Justice, D. (1993). *Case management standards in state community-based long-term care programs for older persons with disabilities*. National Association of State Units on Aging report prepared for the Congressional Research Service.

Kennedy, J., & Litvak, S. (1991). *Case studies of six state personal assistance service programs funded by the Medicaid personal care option*. World Institute on Disability report prepared for Office of the Assistant Secretary for Planning and Evaluation.

Linsk, N., Keigher, S., Simon-Rusinowitz, L., & England., S. (1992). *Wages for caring: Compensating family care of the elderly*. New York: Praeger Press.

Monk, A., & Cox, C. (1989, December). International innovations in home care. *Ageing International, 16*(2), 11-19.

Monk, A., & Cox, C. (1991). *Home care for the elderly*. New York: Auburn House.

Neuschler, E. (1987). *Medicaid eligibility for the elderly in need of long term care*. Center for Policy Research, National Governor's Association.

Organization for Economic Cooperation and Development. (1992). *The care of frail elderly people: Report on policy in Austria*.

Home Care: Moving Forward with Continuous Quality Improvement

Peter W. Shaughnessy, PhD
Robert E. Schlenker, PhD
Kathryn S. Crisler, MS, RN
Angela G. Arnold, MS, RN
Martha C. Powell, PhD
James M. Beaudry, BA

University of Colorado Health Sciences Center
Denver, Colorado

Peter W. Shaughnessy is Professor and Director of the Center for Health Services Research, University of Colorado Health Sciences Center. Robert E. Schlenker is Associate Professor and Associate Director of the Center for Health Services Research; both are faculty members in the University's Department of Medicine. Kathryn S. Crisler and Martha C. Powell are Research Associates and Angela G. Arnold and James M. Beaudry are Professional Research Assistants with the Center for Health Services Research; they are faculty members in the University's School of Nursing.

The research documented here was supported in part by Grant No. 5 RO1 HS08031-02 from the Agency for Health Care Policy and Research; Cooperative Agreement No. 17-C-99051/8-02 and Contract No. 500-88-0054 from the Health Care Financing Administration; and Grant Nos. 13138, 13779, and 19218 from the Robert Wood Johnson Foundation.

Peter W. Shaughnessy can be contacted at the Center for Health Services Research, University of Colorado Health Sciences Center, 1355 S. Colorado Boulevard., Suite 306, Denver, CO 80222.

[Haworth co-indexing entry note]: "Home Care: Moving Forward with Continuous Quality Improvement." Shaughnessy, Peter W. et al. Co-published simultaneously in *Journal of Aging & Social Policy* (The Haworth Press, Inc.) Vol. 7, No. 3/4, 1996, pp. 149-167; and: *From Nursing Homes to Home Care* (ed: Marie E. Cowart and Jill Quadagno) The Haworth Press, Inc., 1996, pp. 149-167. Single or multiple copies of this article are available from The Haworth Document Delivery Service [1-800-342-9678, 9:00 a.m. - 5:00 p.m. (EST)].

SUMMARY. The utility of examining the effectiveness of home care is illustrated by selected examples and applications. The growth rate of home care over the past decade, questions regarding the possibly substantial differences between the quality of home care in rural and urban America, and empirical evidence that suggests inferior quality of home care for health maintenance organization patients support the need for measuring and monitoring outcomes of home care. The conclusions of a research program targeted at developing a system of outcome measures for home care, and the resulting national demonstration program to implement and refine that system, are summarized. *[Article copies available from The Haworth Document Delivery Service: 1-800-342-9678.]*

ISSUES IN QUALITY OF HOME CARE

Increasing Demand for Long-Term Care and Growth of Home Care

The increasing need for long-term care in the United States and its link to our aging population are well-documented. The proportion of persons 65 and older increased from 9.8% of the total population in 1970 to 12.5% of the population in 1990, and is projected to reach 21% to 25% by 2050 (U.S. Bureau of Census, 1992). In addition to the increase in total demand for long-term care services, home care and nursing home providers have experienced substantial increases in patient needs and case-mix complexity over the past decade, resulting in the need not only for more services but also for a more diverse array of services (Shaughnessy & Kramer, 1990).

Within long-term care, home health care is the most rapidly growing sector (Levit, Lazenby, Cowan, & Letsch, 1991). Medicare home health expenditures in 1988 were $2.1 billion, and rose over 500% to $11.0 billion in 1993 (Prospective Payment Assessment Commission, 1994). The growth rate of home health care is outpacing all types of Medicare-covered health care, with projected expenditures expected to increase at an average rate of 10.5% per year through 1999 (National Association for Home Care, 1994). The proportion of total Medicare expenditures spent on home health services increased from 3.8% of Part A expenditures in 1988 to 9.9% in 1992 (ProPAC, 1993) and to 11.5% in 1993 (ProPAC, 1994). Further amplifying the policy significance of home care is the fact that other public funding sources such as Medicaid are experiencing similar growth in expenditures for home and community-based services (Levit et al., 1991; HCFA, 1992). In part, this growth reflects the preference of patients and families to receive health care while remaining in the community whenever possible (the terms "patients," "clients," and "consumers" are used interchangeably).

The Breadth and Depth of Home Care

Home care is defined here as including all professional, paraprofessional, and informal support services provided in the recipient's home (Benjamin, 1992). Formal home care is generally considered to consist of those services provided by a professional or paraprofessional who is paid for the service, whereas informal care typically consists of support and personal care provided in the home by family or friends (termed "home caregivers"). Unlike the nursing home field, where Medicaid and private pay are the dominant payers, Medicare pays for approximately 65% of formal home health care in the United States (Rivlin & Wiener, 1988). The focus here is on patient outcomes resulting from the provision of *formal* home care services, which consist primarily of skilled nursing services, therapy services (physical, occupational, and speech therapy), and medical and social services. These include such highly skilled nursing services as ventilator care, enteral/parenteral feeding, and intravenous (IV) care; others such as wound care; and services provided by physical, occupational, and speech therapists. An important feature of formal home care is training the patient and family in various aspects of self-care. The support services provided by home health aides and other paraprofessionals include assistance with activities of daily living (ADLs), instrumental activities of daily living (IADLs), personal care, and homemaker/chore services.

Conceptualizing and Measuring the Quality of Home Care

It is well-established that quality of care is characterized by and should be defined in terms of a number of dimensions (e.g., Donabedian, 1980; Kane & Kane, 1988; Lohr & Schroeder, 1990; and Shaughnessy, 1989; 1991). Further, there is agreement that quality of care should be measured *ideally* through patient outcomes. However, attributing patient outcomes to care provided is not straightforward. Also, the types of outcomes to assess under different circumstances vary considerably in home care. At times, the most appropriate outcomes include maintaining function, slowing the rate of decline of chronic disease or related conditions, reducing home caregiver stress, or minimizing pain and discomfort prior to death. Avoiding or delaying admission to an institutional care setting can also be regarded as a desirable (utilization) outcome. In contrast, where rehabilitation is possible, outcomes related to improvement in function, restoration to normal living, and compliance with an exercise regimen are appropriate.

Unique features to consider in measuring quality. Unlike institutional long-term care staff, home care providers are guests in the home of the patient. The home environment cannot be controlled or monitored as closely as the patient's environment in an institutional care setting. Relatively routine or episodic problems are more likely to result in exacerbations unless patients and/or home caregivers know how to respond to selected symptoms and circumstances. Teaching patients and families, or increasing awareness of specific issues, is often a critical objective of home care providers. Care coordination with other providers often can be pivotal in attaining optimal patient outcomes.

The unique features of home care affect the manner in which the traditional triad of outcome, process, and structural quality measures can be applied. Outcome measures should be related to specific conditions (through risk adjustment or stratification, or both) that characterize the needs of home care patients served by home care providers. Only then can outcomes be meaningfully linked to care provided by the home care agency when seeking to assess or improve the quality of care. Under such circumstances, process measures, defined in terms of whether and how specific services are provided, can be useful in examining potential causes for differences in outcomes of patients or providers. When outcomes are used to detect problems and, thus, target subsequent investigations of the processes of care for particular types of patients or clients, continuous quality improvement can be attained with greater efficiency (Lohr, 1990).

Current status of outcome measurement. Despite ongoing work to use outcomes in the long-term care field since the early 1980s (summarized in Shaughnessy et al., 1994), no comprehensive approach had emerged by the early 1990s. Several articles have synthesized the available literature on community-based long-term care research (Hedrick & Inui, 1986; Hennessy & Hennessy, 1990; Hughes, 1985; Weissert, Cready, & Pawelak, 1988). Studies of community-based care have included relatively basic outcome measures pertaining to mortality, unmet needs, functional status, quality of life/patient satisfaction, rehospitalization or nursing home placement, and costs. Outcome measures relating to pain, knowledge/compliance, referrals made, caregiver strain, and physiologic or acute conditions for which skilled care is typically provided are less developed. Other studies have focused on frequency of service provision (e.g., Shaughnessy, Schlenker, & Hittle, 1987). None of these studies have focused on a *comprehensive* evaluation of quality, including processes of care linked with a broad range of individual outcome measures. The few published results on home care in rural areas have been based on secondary data (Nyman, Sen, Chan, & Commins, 1991) and characterized by small sample sizes in terms of either patients or agencies (Clinkscale, 1988; Hughes, Conrad, Manheim, & Edelman, 1988; Weissert, Cready, & Pawelak, 1988; Zawadski & Eng, 1988; Zimmer, Groth-Juncker, & McCusker, 1985).

However, more comprehensive measurement approaches to assess home care outcomes for formal services recently have been developed. It now appears feasible to conduct more comprehensive analyses of client- and patient-level outcomes of home care in the United States. Methodologic research indicates that it is possible to move forward with outcome-based quality improvement (OBQI) in the home care field on a preliminary or demonstration basis. By comparing outcomes of home care for a given agency with outcomes for preceding time periods, an approach to continuous quality improvement (CQI) can be developed so that successive annual outcome reports can be used to assess agency progress in influencing patient or client outcomes.

ILLUSTRATIVE FINDINGS

This section presents selected findings from work conducted by the Center for Health Services Research, University of Colorado Health Sciences Center to demonstrate the utility of and need for outcomes assessment in home care. Two sets of results are presented from (1) a small-sample comparison of rural and urban outcomes of home care, and (2) a comparison of outcomes of home care under HMO and fee-for-service payment environments. The findings presented here are not comprehensive, nor are they necessarily representative of quality of care issues and problems nationally. The goal is to highlight the need for and potential value of outcome-based quality improvement.

A Rural-Urban Comparison

Table 1 presents a rural-urban comparison using primary data collected on a longitudinal basis as part of a study to develop outcome measures for home health care. The study was not designed specifically to compare rural and urban patients. Although the rural sample is small (97 patients) and nonrepresentative (three rural communities), Table 1 illustrates the use of outcomes and other types of measures in comparing different groups of patients who receive home health care. Outcome measures are emphasized in this table, and are supplemented by home health care utilization and cost (resource consumption) comparisons. The overall pattern of findings suggests superior outcomes for urban home health care patients. Rural home health patients were hospitalized and received emergent care significantly more often than urban patients. Functional outcomes, based on ADL and IADL measures, consistently favor urban patients (although some differences are statistically insignificant). The physiologic outcomes (based on ordinal scales related to physiologic condition) also suggest better outcomes for urban patients.

The home health utilization measures of visits by discipline suggest different service-use patterns between rural and urban patients, which may be due partly to case-mix differences and variation in available home health resources (e.g., the lack of physical therapists in rural communities). Despite the utilization differences, no significant rural-urban differences emerged in home health cost per patient (i.e., resource consumption). Home health (direct care) minutes per visit differed between rural and urban areas, suggesting that not only the number and mix of visits but also the time per visit may differ between rural and urban areas, which in turn may affect the quality of care.

To adjust for the effect of case-mix differences on outcome differences, logistic regression models were estimated for the following outcomes: hospitalization within three or 12 weeks; improvement pattern in bathing; and discharged improved in bathing. Each logistic regression model included five to nine covariates or risk factors. The results for each model (not shown) increased the magnitude of the urban-rural outcome differences. Although these results are not definitive, they suggest substantial variations in home health patient outcomes between rural and urban locations.

Outcomes Under Capitated and Fee-for-Service Payment Environments

This article reports on a Research Center study designed to compare the cost and quality of home health care between Medicare HMO and fee-for-service (FFS) patients completed in 1994. Two types of Medicare-risk HMO enrollees were studied: those who received home health care from HMO-owned home health agencies and those who received such care under contractual arrangements with Medicare-certified agencies that also provided home care to FFS patients. Analogously, two types of Medicare FFS patients were studied: those who received home health care from contractual agencies that provided care to both HMO and FFS patients,

TABLE 1. Pilot Findings: Illustrative Rural-Urban Outcome and Resource Consumption Profiles[a]

Measures	Means[b] Rural Patients	Urban Patients
Utilization Outcomes		
Hospitalized within 12 Wks of Admission	33.8%	21.6%**
Hospitalized within 3 Wks of Admission	16.2	8.5**
Hospitalized within 3 Wks for Emergent Care	11.8	6.4*
Emergent Care in Outpatient Setting within 3 Wks	4.4	0.7**
Functional Outcomes		
Improvement Pattern in:		
Bathing	29.3%	39.3%*
Feeding	25.0	40.6
Medication Administration	21.4	28.5
Light Meal Preparation	22.7	27.3
Discharged Improved in:		
Bathing	20.0	35.3**
Feeding	10.0	33.3**
Discharged Stabilized in:		
Feeding	63.7	79.2**
Transferring	63.7	78.9**
Medication Administration	64.3	76.8**
Minutes per Visit (by Discipline) During First 3 Wks:		
Skilled Nursing	42.2	47.1
Home Health Aide	62.2	91.1**

Measures	Means[b] Rural Patients	Urban Patients
Physiologic Outcomes		
Improvement Pattern in Depression	40.9%	61.1%*
Improved and Discharged in:		
Number of Pressure Ulcers	12.5	42.4
Discharged Stabilized in:		
Urinary Incontinence	64.9%	82.8%**
Grade of Pressure Ulcers	63.9	82.5**
Home Health Service Use		
Number of Visits by Discipline		
Skilled Nursing	14.7	12.2**
Home Health Aide	3.6	6.1
Physical Therapist	1.4	2.5**
Home Health Resorce Consumption		
Patient-Level Resource Consumption Over 12-Wk Period	$1,477	$1,408
Minutes per Visit (by Discipline) Between the 6th & 9th Wks:		
Skilled Nursing	37.1	46.4**
Home Health Aide	61.2	96.7**

[a]The sample is from a Study to Assess Outcomes of Home Health Care and includes 97 rural patients from 3 agencies and 1,109 urban patients from 31 agencies who were 65 or older at time of admission. For several variables, fewer patients contributed to the above means, since case selection was necessary for some of the outcome variables (e.g., patients who could not improve were excluded from the improvement variables). This can result in a mean difference of a certain size being significant in some cases and not in other cases owing to sample sizes varying by measure.

[b]The designation * denotes $p < .10$, while ** denotes $p < .05$. Significance levels are based on: (1) Fisher's exact test (or its chi-square approximation if expected frequencies permit) for dichotomous variables; or (2) a two-sample Wilcoxon test or t-test for continous or ordinal variables, depending on normality of the underlying distribution using a Kolmorgorov-Smirnov test.

and those who received home health care from agencies that provided care almost exclusively to FFS patients.

Longitudinal primary data on health status and service use were collected on site for a random sample of 1,632 Medicare home health patients from 38 certified home health agencies (9 HMO-owned, 14 contractual HMO/FFS agencies, and 15 "pure-FFS" agencies). Patients were followed from admission until the end of the 12-week study interval, or discharge if it occurred prior to 12 weeks. Data were obtained every three weeks on functional, physiologic, cognitive, and behavioral indicators of health status; home environment and demographics; and service provision and resource consumption. The 12-week or discharge end point was chosen because (1) the study was designed to assess outcomes and costs while patients were under the care of the home health agency, (2) the nature of the Medicare home health benefit typically results in discharge prior to 12 weeks, and (3) attributing outcomes and costs to home health care providers is difficult over longer periods of time after other providers such as hospitals or physicians may have assumed a more prominent role in care management.

Additional details on the study are available in other documents (Shaughnessy, Schlenker, & Hittle 1994, 1995; Shaughnessy et al., 1994; and Schlenker & Shaughnessy, 1995). The main case-mix and utilization/cost findings are highlighted in the next paragraph for contextual purposes. A more comprehensive summary of the outcome findings is presented thereafter.

Overall, the case mix of Medicare FFS patients was more intense than the case mix of Medicare HMO patients in terms of impairments in ADLs, IADLs, and various physiologic conditions. Relative to HMO patients admitted to contractual agencies, HMO patients admitted to HMO-owned agencies were moderately more dependent in terms of ADLs and IADLs. The case mix of patients receiving care from HMO-owned agencies was more heterogeneous than for HMO patients receiving care from contractual agencies. Cost per patient was estimated by summing the products of discipline-specific cost per visit (adjusted for inflation) times the number of visits by each home health discipline for each patient over the study interval. The average cost of home health care per Medicare HMO patient between admission and discharge or 12 weeks (whichever occurred first), unadjusted for case mix, was about two thirds the cost per FFS patient ($877 versus $1,305). Adjusting for case-mix differences and other cost-related factors only reduced the total cost difference from $428 to $401. In all, both before and after case-mix adjustment, the progression in patient-level costs from highest to lowest was: contractual FFS (highest cost), pure-FFS (second highest), contractual HMO (third), and HMO-owned (lowest cost).

The more salient outcome findings are summarized as follows:

- Patient status was measured at multiple points in time in order to examine change in health status over time. Outcome findings were risk-adjusted to compensate for the case-mix differences noted previously. Distinct patterns of outcome differences were found in comparisons of Medicare HMO patients with Medicare FFS patients (pooled comparisons). First, the overall profiles of outcomes showed significantly more favorable outcomes for FFS patients than for HMO patients. When significant differences occurred for individual outcome measures, risk-adjusted outcomes tended to be superior for FFS patients. In fact, no risk-adjusted 12-week outcomes were superior for HMO patients. FFS patients exhibited significantly superior outcomes for 14 of the 55 different 12-week patient-status outcome measures. For example, the risk-adjusted mean improvement in the ADL of "eating" (i.e., ability to feed oneself) was 14.3 percentage points greater for FFS patients: 33.9% of HMO patients compared with 48.2% of FFS patients improved in eating disabilities (analyses were restricted to those patients who had eating disabilities at admission).
- Relative to contractual HMO patients, the overall outcome profiles again demonstrated a pattern of significantly better outcomes for contractual FFS patients. Further, contractual FFS patients had superior risk-adjusted outcomes for 17 of the 12-week outcome measures (and an inferior outcome for only one such measure). For example, the risk-adjusted mean difference for the outcome of "discharged to independent living *and* stabilized in the ability to manage oral medications" was 9.6 percentage points greater for FFS patients (71.0% of contractual HMO patients compared with 80.6% of contractual FFS patients).
- Comparing HMO patients admitted to HMO-owned agencies with FFS patients admitted to agencies that contract very little with HMOs (i.e., pure-FFS agencies) resulted in the same overall pattern of better outcomes for FFS patients. Outcomes were also compared between the two types of HMO patients, with the general finding that some outcomes were superior for contractual HMO patients relative to HMO patients admitted to HMO-owned agencies.
- Outcome comparisons by strata or patient type generally substantiated the above findings. For example, the same overall patterns of superior outcomes for FFS patients were apparent when analyses

were restricted separately to patients admitted to home care from hospitals, patients admitted from the community, those with rehabilitation care needs, patients with mental and behavioral impairments, cardiac patients, patients with at least moderate recovery potential, those with a below-average need for personal care services, those with an above-average need for such services, patients with above-average functional impairments, and patients with below-average functional impairments. FFS versus HMO outcomes were not different for wound care patients, however.

Since the cost analyses for the study found progressively lower cost per episode for contractual FFS patients, FFS patients admitted to pure-FFS agencies, contractual HMO patients, and HMO patients admitted to HMO-owned agencies, and since the general pattern of superiority in outcomes follows this same sequence, it appears that a volume-outcome relationship exists that points to a positive association between utilization/cost per episode and patient-status outcomes in the home health care field.

The findings that have emerged suggest that further attention should be devoted: (1) to reassessing managed care practices that may be overly restrictive in terms of the use of home health care services; (2) to identifying situations of overprovision of home care services in the FFS sector for which little or no improvement in patient outcomes is obtained; and (3) as a consequence of both (1) and (2), to developing OBQI approaches for home care.

DEVELOPMENT OF OUTCOME MEASURES AND THE OBQI APPROACH

The preceding findings illustrate the need for and value of investigating and assessing patient outcomes of home care (in view of patient needs). They also illustrate some of the factors to consider in assessing outcomes and support the need for a practical system of outcome measures for home care. In this section, the Center for Health Services Research's program to develop outcome measures for quality improvement purposes is discussed.

In 1989, a six-year study was undertaken to provide a framework for OBQI in home health care. The study's results, approaches, and conclusions are summarized here. From its inception, the purpose of this program was to develop, test, and refine a system of outcome measures that could be used for OBQI in home care agencies. This measure system was intended to form the foundation of an approach to CQI that could be used to enhance care in agencies where quality (measured by using patient outcomes) is found to be lacking, and to reinforce quality in agencies where care is found to be exemplary. This would be accomplished through the use of agency-specific outcome profiles that can be compared with statistical norms based on data from multiple agencies or from a given agency's outcome profiles for previous time periods.

Developing the quality measures that would constitute this system was challenging. The objective was to specify a comprehensive system of measures that would be of value to home care consumers, providers, regulators, and payers. This is a different challenge from that encountered in many research and evaluation efforts because the measure system is to be used for a more pervasive purpose than examining a single approach (i.e., evaluate a particular program) or specific issue at a point in time. Endeavoring to attain the goal of implementing a practical approach to OBQI required that the quality measures satisfy several criteria, including but not restricted to: reliability, clinical acceptability, precision of measurement, minimal burden for the type of application required, ease or practicality of risk adjustment, agency-level variation, minimal potential for gameability, minimal redundancy among measures, acceptability by the industry for quality improvement purposes, and, as a comprehensive system, the capacity to be revised or improved over time and to contribute to CQI at both the agency and system levels. Practically speaking, it was apparent from the outset that those criteria could not be satisfied perfectly.

The intent was to balance practical considerations with a need to be comprehensive and systematic in investigating measures that are useful for quality improvement in home care. Toward this end, the Research Center attempted to develop a parsimonious system of measures that has evolved from first reviewing an array of measures and measurement approaches, data sources, and data collection methods. To err in the direction of being overly comprehensive in the early stages of the project was viewed as lessening the likelihood of omitting important concepts, measures, past work, and practical approaches to quality assurance. Over the course of the study various measurement approaches were refined. The total number of measures was reduced. It is important to emphasize, however, that the final measure set will continue to undergo refinement and should not be viewed as static. Even over the several years that the study was conducted, it was apparent that several measures appropriate in the late 1980s would need to be replaced by others more appropriate in the mid 1990s–simply because of changes in home care, case mix of home care agencies, and the changes in service provision that occurred over this period.

After an initial feasibility phase, the empirical phase of the study began in mid-1991 and continued through 1994. This involved analyzing primary longitudinal data that were collected on 3,427 patients from 49 home health agencies (44 certified and 5 noncertified) throughout the United States. Data were collected at start of care and 30-day intervals after the start of care, up to 90 days or until the patient was discharged from the home health agency. The data items and quality measures that underwent testing and refinement in the empirical phase were those that were specified as a result of the initial developmental and feasibility components of the project.

In the previous studies mentioned in this article, various approaches to outcome measurement were developed and tested. In this research program to develop a system of quality measures for home care, the more useful approaches have involved improvement/stabilization measures, which are dichotomies indicating whether a given patient-status scale reflects improvement or nonworsening/stabilization between the initial and final points in time at which the client is studied. Additional outcome measures found to be useful are dichotomies indicating whether a client is admitted to a hospital, receives emergent care (i.e., an unscheduled emergency room visit), is admitted to a nursing home, or is discharged *and* stabilized in terms of various measures of health status. A variety of different approaches were tested with similar results.[1]

Figure 1 illustrates the outcome taxonomy used in the study, and also includes process and structural dimensions of the quality of care. (Although *process quality measures* were developed and refined on this study and *structural quality measures* pertaining to characteristics of the provider or the community environment in which care is delivered were examined, they are not presented here since outcome measures were the focus of the study.)

Figure 2 shows the classification system for focused outcome measures developed as part of this project. The Quality Indicator Group (QUIG) system of patient conditions was constructed to develop measures of the quality of home care. It was developed over a period of several years so that quality measures (both outcome and process measures) would apply (nearly) uniformly for most patients belonging to a given QUIG, but would be heterogenous across QUIGs. Assignment to QUIGs occurs based on medical diagnoses (e.g., diabetes mellitus); treatment goals (e.g., rehabilitation conditions); occasionally, certain therapeutic interventions (e.g., infusion therapy); stage of disease (e.g., terminal conditions); and related variables. The classification system was developed conceptually following a review of classification systems used in home health care and related health care settings (Kramer, Shaughnessy, Bauman, & Crisler, 1990), and subjected to multiple reviews by home care clinicians who concentrated on the utility of the system for specifying focused outcome

FIGURE 1. Taxonomy Used for Measures of the Quality of Home Health Care

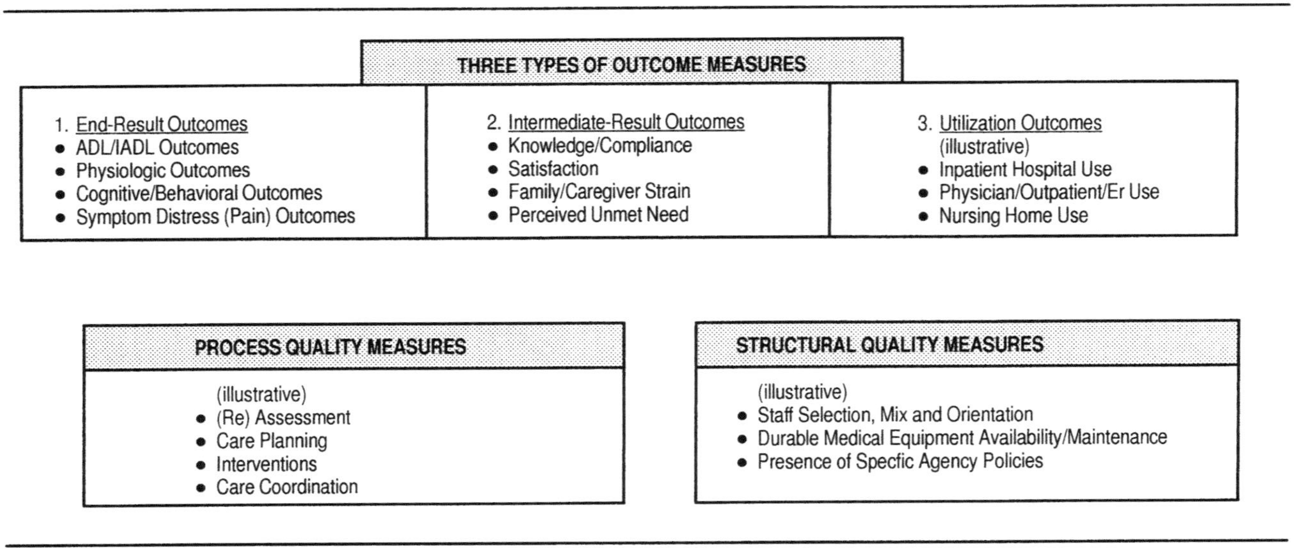
THREE TYPES OF OUTCOME MEASURES
1. End-Result Outcomes
• ADL/IADL Outcomes
• Physiologic Outcomes
• Cognitive/Behavioral Outcomes
• Symptom Distress (Pain) Outcomes
2. Intermediate-Result Outcomes
• Knowledge/Compliance
• Satisfaction
• Family/Caregiver Strain
• Perceived Unmet Need
3. Utilization Outcomes
(illustrative)
• Inpatient Hospital Use
• Physician/Outpatient/Er Use
• Nursing Home Use
PROCESS QUALITY MEASURES
(illustrative)
• (Re) Assessment
• Care Planning
• Interventions
• Care Coordination
STRUCTURAL QUALITY MEASURES
(illustrative)
• Staff Selection, Mix and Orientation
• Durable Medical Equipment Availability/Maintenance
• Presence of Specfic Agency Policies

measures and process quality measures that pertain to each QUIG. An instrument was developed to classify patients into QUIGs, and the stratification approach was field-tested and refined twice.

The QUIG system covers all adult home care patients, and a patient can be classified into several QUIGs. The QUIGs are subdivided into acute and chronic categories. The acute category covers unstable conditions requiring skilled care and acute exacerbations of chronic problems; the treatment plan may require frequent review and modification for such conditions. The patient's health status or ability to provide self-care is expected to improve (except in the case of acute terminal conditions, Group 13 in Figure 2). The chronic category covers long-term or stable conditions requiring skilled and/or unskilled care, primarily for the maintenance of functioning or prevention of further deterioration or complications, not typically requiring frequent changes in the treatment plan. The QUIG approach is being used so that focused outcome quality measures can be analyzed on a QUIG-specific basis. QUIGs are also used as case-mix measures or risk factors in analyzing global outcome measures (see later material). Process quality measures can also be analyzed for particular QUIGs and used to further examine reasons for QUIG-specific outcome differences. However, other classification systems can also be used, depending on the application.

The outcome measures are termed either "global" or "focused" depending on whether they pertain to all clients or specific client groups selected for the purposes of lessening the need to risk-adjust within groups. Global measures include end-result outcomes such as improvement and stabilization in ambulation and improvement in ability to manage oral medications. Global utilization outcome measures include acute hospitalization and emergent care (possibly for specific reasons). Focused measures for cardiac and peripheral vascular conditions include improvement in dyspnea, stabilization in weight, improvement in activity level, and emergent care for cardiac problems.

As a result of the research described here, a two-tiered system of outcome measures was developed as the basis for individual agencies and payers to monitor and improve the effectiveness of home health care. Specific measures and associated data items were recommended for use so that patient outcomes reflecting changes (or no changes) in health status between the admission of a client and follow up, as well as utilization outcomes such as hospitalization, emergent care, and nursing home admission can be aggregated across patients to the agency level, thereby permitting an analysis of agency performance in terms of the effectiveness of care.

FIGURE 2. Taxonomy of Patient Conditions for Focused Quality Measures

ACUTE CONDITIONS

Rehabilitation Conditions	Medical Conditions	Specialized Care	Other Acute
1. Orthopedic 2. Neuromuscular	3. Cardiac/Peripheral Vascular 4. Pulmonary 5. Diabetes Mellitus 6. Gastrointestinal Disorders 7. Contagious/Communicable	8. Oxygen Therapy 9. IV/Infusion Therapy 10. Enteral/Parenteral Nutrition Therapy 11. Ventilator	12. Open Wounds/Lesions 13. Terminal Conditions 14. Urinary Incontinence/ Catheters 15. Mental/Emotional

CHRONIC CONDITIONS

1. Dependence in Living Skills 2. Dependence in Personal Care 3. Impaired Ambulation/Mobility	4. Eating Disability 5. Urinary Incontinence/Catheter Use 6. Dependence in Medication Administration	7. Chronic Pain 8. Cognitive/Mental/Behavioral Probs. 9. Chronic Patients: Caregiver Present

A two-stage quality improvement screen was recommended, in which the first-stage screen is based on patient outcomes. Either exemplary or inferior outcomes can trigger a second-stage screen to investigate processes of care that would result in reinforcement or remediation of care behaviors. Patient-specific data necessary to outcome measures would be collected by agency care providers at admission and every 60 days until discharge. The first tier of outcome measures (and data items) termed the "core measures," would constitute a payer-required set of measures that would be computed for all patients. For example, the Medicare program might use this core set to construct outcome profiles for individual agencies that subsequently could be utilized in the Medicare certification process, possibly replacing other more process- and structural-based features of this program. State Medicaid agencies could use the approach to accumulate comparable uniform longitudinal databases to monitor the case mix and outcomes of their home or community care programs. Home care agencies could elect to implement an OBQI system at the agency level with a more comprehensive set of measures than the Medicare or Medicaid systems. These comprehensive measures, termed "full-scope measures," include the core measures as a subset and permit a more detailed analysis of outcomes for those agencies interested in implementing a more in-depth approach to OBQI.[2] The OBQI approach is currently being refined under the national Medicare Home Health Quality Assurance and Improvement Demonstration. The demonstration will involve 50 agencies nationwide in implementing, testing, and improving the OBQI approach over a four-and-a-half-year period.

COMMENTS

Considerable information is collected and generated by home care agencies for several purposes, including quality improvement, management, billing, patient reporting, and record-keeping for the purposes of documenting patient care and patient assessment. Since we are currently undergoing substantial changes in home care in this country, an exceptional opportunity exists. As we move forward with and hopefully enhance our ability to measure the effectiveness of home care, a framework that focuses first on outcomes and secondly on processes of care should prove useful. However, the need for information to support such a system is substantial. As we change the data systems necessary to provide, regulate, and finance home care, we should do so with a view toward measuring outcomes. A carefully designed core system of data items which constitute the prerequisites for measuring outcomes is essential. A parsimonious set of such items should be collected uniformly by providers of home care–for all clients, as part of the patient/client assessment process. Such data should be collected at regular intervals, such as at admission and every 60 days thereafter until and including discharge. Outcome reports can be generated based on such data. An agency's outcome profile can be compared to aggregate profiles from other agencies throughout the country and to an outcome profile for its preceding time period, thereby forming the basis for continuous quality improvement. If an agency's performance warrants it, the outcome profiles can be succeeded by abstracting information from patient records or by a less formal means of examining care/services provided (the second-stage or process quality screen) to assess reasons for inferior or exemplary performance. The infrastructure–in terms of regulatory, financing, and agency-level involvement needed to support OBQI in home care–will be specified and revised over the course of the next few years, as part of the national Home Health Quality Assurance and Improvement Demonstration.

ENDNOTES

1. These different approaches include Markov-chain transitions; length or percentage of time until the client is in an improved or worsened state; patterns of improvement, stabilization or worsening; and change in various aggregate indicators of health status.

2. Implementing a large-scale OBQI system based on a wide array of measures and data items can be expensive and burdensome if attempted at a single point in time. Consequently, except in those instances where mandated (and possibly financed, at least indirectly) by a payer or when an agency has the resources to do so, we recommend a phased approach. Agencies should begin with selected outcome measures, possibly for specific patient or client types, and with a relatively small set of data items. Thereafter, as experience is gained and familiarity with the approach increases, additional patient/client types, measures, and data items can be added until a full-scope system is in place and the same data items are used for purposes of assessment and outcome measurement.

REFERENCES

Benjamin, A.E. (1992). An overview of in-home health and supportive services for older persons. In M. Ory & A. Duncker (Eds.), *In-home care for older people: Health and supportive services* (pp. 9-52). Newbury Park, CA: Sage Publications.

Clinkscale, R.M. (1988). *National evaluation: Medicaid section 2176 home and community care waivers*. Medicaid Program Evaluation Working Paper 1.15.

Washington, DC: Health Care Financing Administration, U.S. Department of Health and Human Services.

Donabedian, A. (1980). *Explorations in quality assessment and monitoring, Volume 1: The definition of quality and approaches to its assessment*. Ann Arbor, MI: Health Administration Press.

Health Care Financing Administration, U.S. Department of Health and Human Services. (1992, September). *1992 HCFA Statistics*. (HCFA Publication No. 03333). Baltimore, MD: Bureau of Data Management and Strategy, HCFA.

Hedrick, S.C., & Inui, T.S. (1986). The effectiveness and cost of home care: An information synthesis. *Health Services Research*, *20*(6), 851-880.

Hennessy, C.H., & Hennessy, M. (1990). Community-based long-term care for the elderly: Evaluation practice reconsidered. *Medical Care Review*, *47*(2), 221-259.

Hughes, S.L. (1985). Apples and oranges? A review evaluation of community-based long-term care. *Health Services Research*, *20*(4), 261-287.

Hughes, S.L., Conrad, K.J., Manheim, L.M., & Edelman, P.L. (1988). Impact of long-term home care on mortality, functional status, and unmet needs. *Health Services Research*, *23*(2), 269-294.

Kane, R.A., & Kane, R.L. (1988). Long-term care: Variations on a quality assurance theme. *Inquiry*, *25*(1), 132-146.

Kramer, A.M., Shaughnessy, P.W., Bauman, M.K., & Crisler, K.S. (1990). Assessing and assuring the quality of home health care: A conceptual framework. *Milbank Quarterly*, *68*(3), 413-443.

Levit, K.R., Lazenby, H.C., Cowan, C.A.,& Letsch, S.W. (1991). National health expenditures, 1990. *Health Care Financing Review*, *13*(1), 29-54.

Lohr, K.N. (Ed.) (1990). *Medicare: A strategy for quality assurance, Volume I.* Washington, DC: National Academy Press.

Lohr, K.N., & Schroeder, S.A. (1990). A strategy for quality assurance in Medicare. *New England Journal of Medicine*, *322*(10), 707-712.

National Association for Home Care. (1994, March 11). Medicare home care and hospice programs continue rapid growth. *NAHC Report* (553), 6-7.

Nyman, J.A., Sen, A., Chan, B.Y., & Commins, P.P. (1991). Urban/rural differences in home health patients and services. *The Gerontologist*, *31*(4), 457-466.

Prospective Payment Assessment Commission. (1993, June 11). *Medicare and the American Health Care System: Report to Congress*, Part 2, Number 751. Chicago, IL: Commerce Clearing House, Inc.

Prospective Payment Assessment Commission. (1994, June 9). *Medicare and the American health care system: Report to Congress*, Part 2, Number 805. Chicago, IL: Commerce Clearing House, Inc.

Rivlin, A.M., & Wiener, J.M., with Hanley, R.J., & Spence, D.A. (1988). *Caring for the disabled elderly: Who will pay*? Washington, DC: The Brookings Institution.

Schlenker, R.E., Shaughnessy, P.W., & Hittle, D.F. (1995, Fall). Patient-level cost of home health care under capitated and fee-for-service payment. *Inquiry*, *32*(3).

Shaughnessy, P.W. (1989). Quality of nursing home care: Problems and pathways. *Generations*, *13*(1), 17-20.

Shaughnessy, P.W. (1991). *Shaping policy for long-term care: Learning from the effectiveness of hospital swing beds*. Ann Arbor, MI: Health Administration Press.

Shaughnessy, P.W., Crisler, K.S., Schlenker, R.E., Arnold, A.G., Kramer, A.M., Powell, M.C., & Hittle, D.F. (1994, Fall). Measuring and assuring the quality of home care. *Health Care Financing Review*, *16*(1), 35-68.

Shaughnessy, P.W., & Kramer, A.M. (1990). The increased needs of patients in nursing homes and patients receiving home health care. *New England Journal of Medicine*, *322*(1), 21-27.

Shaughnessy, P.W., Schlenker, R.E., & Hittle, D.F. (1987). *An evaluation study of the national swing-bed program in the 1980s*. Denver, CO: Center for Health Services Research, University of Colorado Health Sciences Center.

Shaughnessy, P.W., Schlenker, R.E., & Hittle, D.F. (1994, Fall). Home health care outcomes under capitated and fee-for-service payment. *Health Care Financing Review*, *16*(1), 187-222.

Shaughnessy, P.W., Schlenker, R.E., Hittle, D.F., with Kramer, A.M., Crisler, K.S., Spencer, M.J., DeVore, P.A., Grant, W.V., Beaudry, J.M., & Chandramouli, V. (1994, February). *Study of home health care quality and cost under capitated and fee-for-service payment systems. Volume 2: Technical Report*. Denver, CO: Center for Health Policy Research.

Shaughnessy, P.W., Schlenker, R.E., & Hittle, D.F. (1995, April). Case mix of home health patients under capitated and fee-for-service payment. *Health Services Research*, *30*(1), 79-113.

U.S. Bureau of the Census. (1992). *Current population reports, special studies: Sixty-five plus in America* (pp. 23-178). Washington, DC: U.S. Government Printing Office.

Weissert, W.G., Matthews Cready, C., & Pawelak, J.E. (1988). Past and future of home and community-based long-term care. *Milbank Quarterly*, *66*(2), 309-388.

Zawadski, R.T., & Eng, C. (1988). Case management in capitated long-term care. *Health Care Financing Review*, Annual Supplement, 75-81.

Zimmer, J., Groth-Juncker, A., & McCusker, J. (1985). A randomized controlled study of a home health care team. *American Journal of Public Health*, *75*(20), 134-141.

Long-Term Care Policy and the American Family

Marie E. Cowart, DrPH

Florida State University
Tallahassee, Florida

SUMMARY. This article examines current and proposed long-term care policies and the social values of American families by looking at the influence of policy on family behavior. The analysis asks two questions. First, have our policies in recent years supported or undermined family values regarding the care of older members? Second, are our existing family values compatible with home and community-based long-term care reform proposals? Aaron, Mann, and Taylor's (1994) model for policy and changing values provides direction throughout. Findings based on behavior as a proxy for values suggest that current policies influence family values, and in turn, family values influence policies. Future policy is discussed in light of changed values, American family structure, dysfunctional families, individualism and collectivism, and gender neutrality and justice. *[Article copies available from The Haworth Document Delivery Service: 1-800-342-9678.]*

Marie E. Cowart is Professor at the Pepper Institute on Aging and Public Policy and the Department of Urban and Regional Planning at Florida State University. She is also an Editor of this volume.

Dr. Cowart wishes to express her appreciation to her colleagues who commented on an earlier version of this paper: Rebecca Miles-Doan, Jill Quadagno, Lynn Sittig, and Linda Vinton, as well as to two anonymous reviewers.

The author can be contacted care of the Pepper Institute on Aging and Public Policy, Florida State University, Tallahassee, FL 32306.

[Haworth co-indexing entry note]: "Long-Term Care Policy and the American Family." Cowart, Marie E. Co-published simultaneously in *Journal of Aging & Social Policy* (The Haworth Press, Inc.) Vol. 7, No. 3/4, 1996, pp. 169-184; and: *From Nursing Homes to Home Care* (ed: Marie E. Cowart and Jill Quadagno) The Haworth Press, Inc., 1996, pp. 169-184. Single or multiple copies of this article are available from The Haworth Document Delivery Service [1-800-342-9678, 9:00 a.m. - 5:00 p.m. (EST)].

As our population has aged over the last 30 years, the need for a comprehensive long-term care policy has become more urgent than when Medicare and Medicaid were passed in 1965 to help with the needs of poor and older Americans. Developed incrementally, what long-term care policies we have now provide limited nursing home days and home health care coverage for everyone over age 65, and institutional nursing home care for those meeting financial-eligibility screens. While much research is directed to financing long-term care, little attention has been paid to the effect of our long-term care policies on the American family.

Although the support for governmental growth and expansion that existed when national health policy (i.e., Medicare and Medicaid) was first adopted is gone, dramatic policy change for long-term care is found in President Clinton's 1994 health reform proposal. The policies of the 1990s are developing in an atmosphere that calls for less federal debt, fairness for a pluralistic population, and a sense of duty and caring for others, but that is experiencing widespread dysfunctional behavior (Aaron, Mann, & Taylor, 1994; Yankelovich, 1994). This article asks two questions. First, have the long-term care policies that we do have shaped family values by supporting or by undermining traditional values about one's obligation to provide care for older family members? Second, are existing family values compatible with proposals for home and community-based long-term care reform?

Values and attitudes shape many aspects of life. Regarding care and aging, social norms shape choices in caregiving practices, end-of-life decisions, and family relations. They may emerge from lessons taught by family, friends, and community (Aaron, Mann, & Taylor, 1994). Henry Aaron and colleagues (1994) use this perspective to develop a model for value modification that includes these five dimensions: economic incentives or direct policy influences, learning that occurs during childrearing, correcting knowledge misperceptions with education, persuasion by public figures, and value formation learned from the local community. They and others acknowledge that value explanations are less explicit than other measures, but that there is good reason to examine values since examining policies can illuminate basic social values and the relation of family values to policy (Kingson, Hirshorn, & Cronman, 1986).

In this article, the definition of values emerges from personal utility or usefulness. Values refer to those ideals or aspirations family members hold in esteem (Ladd, 1976)–because of their usefulness. Examples of family values include an emphasis on family life including and beyond the nuclear family, caring beyond one's self, a sense of pragmatism about the future, an acceptance of the blurring family roles, and the need for family bonds, obligations, and shared consumption. Family values are nested in individual and social values. As individuals, Americans value choice, independence, human freedom, and competitiveness. In the past, there was a greater emphasis on social values of collectiveness and community, whereas now, particularly since the 1950s, values of individualism, equity, accepting diversity, and facing up to government's role and the economy are held (Popenoe, 1994).

This shift in emphasis on collectiveness and the social order to one of individualism has emerged in part from an emphasis on competitiveness and economic success (Popenoe, 1994). We now experience an emphasis on market productivity, or "exchange value," rather than "use value," which emphasizes a decent life for all (Hendricks & Leedham, 1991); this results in individuals and individual families putting more emphasis on autonomy for the individual family members. The influence of use value can compensate for the conflicting emphasis on productivity that has pervaded the U.S. health and long-term care industries and strengthened the impact of interest-group politics. In health and long-term care policy formulation, this shift in emphasis may be viewed as a tension between the exchange values of production represented in the policy arena by interest groups and the family values of human welfare that are represented in the polling place.

We can assume that individual values change as a result of learning from parents and exposure to family role models, and that societal values change as social priorities change (Bayles, 1987). Societal-level value concerns include value conflicts, lack of a unified consensus on social values, and an absence of prevailing values among the dysfunctional components of society (Aaron et al., 1994). There are times when individuals consider both personal values and social values (Bayles, 1987).

Because values are not easily available for examination or measurement, this author uses behavior as an observable proxy indicator for prevailing family values. While behaviors may not always accurately reflect normative or prevailing values, especially when value conflicts underlie choices of behaviors (Ladd, 1976), they can provide valuable insights into values and their relationships to policy (Aaron et al., 1994).

INFLUENCE OF POLICY ON FAMILY VALUES AND LONG-TERM CARE

Have our existing long-term care policies shaped family values by supporting or undermining values regarding the care of older family members? Daniel Yankelovich (1994) reminds us that the atmosphere surrounding the passage of Medicare and Medicaid included economic growth and a sense of affluence riding the wave of excessive hospital beds funded by the post-World War II Hill-Burton Act.[1] Families lived with hope for the future and a "better life" for their children. Achieving an education and acquiring material goods were highly valued. Other than the family, the major options for long-term care were the local nursing home or home health services provided by public, voluntary, not-for-profit, or singly owned for-profit agencies at affordable costs for many persons (Harrington, Newcomer, & Estes, 1985; Kane & Kane, 1987). The smaller numbers of frail and disabled elders and shorter life expectancy than today (Atchley, 1994; Serow, Sly, and Wrigley, 1990) contributed less to a concern for long-term care than to a felt need to enhance acute care by developing "high tech" care centers, and new diagnostic and treatment approaches. Several policy landmarks serve to illustrate their influence on observed family behavior in making caregiving choices.

A simple example is the effect of certificate of need policy[2] on limiting nursing home beds. This policy, which may be viewed as a social solution to the emphasis on exchange values and the overproduction of health services, contributed to high nursing home bed occupancy (91.5% in 1991) and even waiting times for admissions (Harrington, Newcomer, & Estes, 1985; Kane & Kane, 1987; NCHS, 1994), shifting care to alternate resources, among which was the informal care provided by family members.

In another instance, the financial eligibility restrictions for Medicaid resulted in private payment for much nursing home care. Currently, over half the cost of nursing home care is paid out of pocket (Wiener, Illston, & Hanley, 1994), causing nursing home charges to be paid largely from family rather than public resources. The high cost of nursing home care results in an accompanying spend-down effect for families: (1) the individual family member needing nursing home care becomes eligible for Medicaid funding, or (2) families may move their frail or disabled family member from nursing home care to less costly alternatives, often informal care provided by family members. In a 1993 poll, 68% of women and 64% of men reported that long-term care costs were a major concern for the future[3] (Gallup & Saad, 1993).

Even existing acute care policies serve as incentives to reinforce family caregiving. A good example is the transition of cataract surgery from an inpatient procedure before 1980 to an almost exclusively outpatient experience. This has been activated by expanded technology, concerns for reductions in health costs, and Professional Service Review Organization policies (Davis, Anderson, Rowland, & Steinberg, 1990; Kane & Kane,

1987). Formerly, when cataract surgery was an inpatient procedure, care of the family member was the responsibility of hospital personnel and the patient went home when convalescence was complete. Although the shift to outpatient surgery occurred primarily as a cost-containment measure, it stimulated families and friends to assume responsibility for an individual's activities of daily living, if only temporarily. In this instance, family caregiving is reinforced by the change in policy from inpatient to outpatient surgical care.

Home health care provides another example. Medicare home health regulations allow reimbursement for teaching a family member to care for their sick or disabled members (Garvey & Logue, 1988). This policy provides a direct incentive to shift the responsibility for care from the formal paid system to the informal family system. For families wanting to care for their disabled members at home, this policy supports their informal caregiving.

Policies have shifted the function of many nursing homes from residential facilities to temporary convalescent and rehabilitative centers. Two influences have contributed to this change–the Medicare Prospective Payment system for hospital care and Medicare limits on the number of nursing home days covered. The first has shortened hospital length of stay by shifting medically stable patients into the nursing home for convalescence, while the second limits the days of nursing home care that are fully or even partially reimbursed. These incentives stimulate families to arrange alternate forms of care and individuals to engage in self-help rehabilitative activities rather than view the nursing home admission as an end-of-life experience (Florida Health Care Cost Containment Board, 1987; 1994). Such policies can support family caregiving of their elder members and reinforce their elder's autonomy and independence or individualism.

Policies governing when nursing home residents become eligible for Medicaid reimbursement influence families to shelter income and assets so that Medicaid eligibility can occur without the family estate being completely voided (Binstock, 1993). Despite policies from OBRA 1993 requiring a three-year financial history and enforcement procedure, if financial transfers are done early, no questions are asked. Since Medicaid eligibility varies by state, it is not uncommon to see interstate migration to the state where adult children reside when nursing home admission is imminent (Litwak & Longino, 1987; Longino & Crown, 1990). These policies foster the involvement of families with their elder members and reinforce family solidarity, although it is unknown whether such behavior is due to the policy or a concern for the adult children's future inheritance.

Other dimensions of Aaron's (1994) model (child rearing, correcting misconceptions, persuasion, and the influence of local institutions) also affect family behavior and long-term care–some examples are worth mentioning. When family caregiving occurs in the home, the home environment can teach children about helping family members–a lesson that may carry over into adulthood when the next generation of parental caregiving responsibilities arise. The altering of misconceptions concerning long-term care by public figures through education or persuasion occurs irregularly, and educational policies and local organizations do little to provide knowledge about available service networks to support family caring for their disabled members. Members of groups such as the American Association of Retired Persons (AARP) can learn about long-term care issues through their publications. In a 1994 Gallup poll[3] (Moore, 1994) that asked about the top health benefits which poll respondents would want guaranteed, almost half listed "nursing home care" as their first or second choice. Whether this choice was made because of fear of financial ruin or to assure protection of the potential family caregiver's time, many families learn about the long-term care system only when the need arises and the time for planning has passed.

Although these examples show how policies can be reflected in family behavior, they may not be the only influence. Other factors contribute to caregiving arrangements. Some indirect policy influences include less poverty among the aged because of income security (Ball, 1994), more elders living in their own households (U.S. Bureau of the Census, 1992), increased life expectancy (Serow, Sly, & Wrigley, 1990), longer active life expectancy resulting in a healthier, older population (Fries, 1980), and access to regular care afforded by widespread Medicare coverage (Doty, 1992). With these and other social changes, families have adapted traditional caregiving that took place in the household by adult children and members of the extended family (Hareven, 1992) to caregiving models which have developed because of the improved health of elders and that fact that families often live in separate households. Two such variations are long-distance caregiving and the proliferation of free-standing case management services for those elderly whose families live in a distant geographic location (Monk, 1988). These changes in caregiving patterns may represent a shift in caregiving practices, or they may simply represent ways families cope with the conflicts of having the responsibilities for work and their primary family in one locality and their parents in another.

FAMILY VALUES AND THE FUTURE LONG-TERM CARE POLICY

The first part of this article discussed the relationship between our long-term care policies and family behavior from the 1960s to the present. Because our arrangements and our policies concerning long-term care are likely to change, this section of the article reviews informal elder care and the relationship of families and long-term care policy proposals for the future.

The major thrust of any proposal for long-term care will likely emphasize the use of federal funds for programs designed and managed by the states to reimburse home and community-based services for severely disabled persons of all ages, thus universalizing access to long-term care and minimizing age segregation. Emphasizing home and community-based care implies a continued emphasis on the support of informal systems of care. While these proposals will be compatible with keeping people at home, which the elderly prefer, and with the aims of traditional nuclear and extended families, they may be ineffective in some instances. Two considerations are the changing structure of the American family and the apparent increase in vulnerable populations. Another potential for conflict arises from a growing emphasis on individualism rather than collectivism.

Current Family Structure. Although under any new long-term care plan there will be a continued or increased reliance on informal caregiving, many family structures are not optimal for the informal caregiving that is a basic assumption of home and community-based care. Increased life expectancy has resulted in more generations being available today to care for the disabled, although lower fertility and birth rates as an expression of individualism have reduced the number of household members who are available as caregivers. Lower fertility and birth rates will also contribute to more elders and disabled having only one child, or who are childless, thus reducing the number of available caregivers. Increased divorce rates confound family relationships and responsibilities for caregiving. From 1970 to 1983, the number of single-parent households grew by 69% (Wisensale, 1988). Half of all children live in one-parent households (U.S. Census, 1992). Changing family structures and childlessness will leave some disabled elders without family supports, and may burden some adult children with the caregiving responsibility of more than one parent or stepparent.

The future also suggests increases in the total elderly population and the number of elderly living alone. In the three decades 1960 to 1990, the percentage of elders living alone increased; in particular, women and black men have higher rates of solo living arrangements than do white males.

Furthermore, elders without living family members have higher nursing home admission rates than those with them (Doty, 1986).

The increasing number of teen pregnancies–again an expression of individualism–foretells a scenario of the oldest old being cared for by their 60- to 70-year-old children. At the same time, women who choose to delay childbirth until the third decade will likely have the dual responsibilities of childcare and eldercare (Bengston, 1993; Wisensale, 1988).

However, Robyn Stone and Peter Kemper (1989) add a more salutary dimension to the concern for adults in nontraditional family structures assuming caregiving responsibilities. They point out that women who engage in childrearing while they provide care to older relatives comprise 0.6% of the women with children under age 15 (n = 164,000). They compare this with the 4.2 million employed women and 163,000 working men who provide primary care for children under the age of six. Employed primary caregivers for the elderly make up 0.3% of men and 1.3% of women employed full time (30+ hours weekly). The larger group is the 2.6 million primary caregivers of spouses or parents who are not employed or responsible for childcare. Stone and Kemper hasten to add that though the number of caregivers with work or childrearing responsibilities is relatively small, this does not diminish the stress or sense of duty these persons assume. Seven percent of U.S. adults are spouses or children of disabled elders, with the 45- to 54-year-old group providing the most care. Stone and Kemper emphasize that in planning long-term care reform, the 13.3 million potential and active caregivers and the 4.4 million disabled adults needing care must be considered.

Since most caregiving responsibilities fall to female family members (Stone, Cafferata, & Sangl, 1986), the increased labor-force participation rates of women, particularly minority women from 1960 to 1990, cause one to ask if greater reliance on home and community-based services will increase caregiver stress, or whether it will provide more access to formal services and reduce caregiver burden. The emphasis on home and community-based services will continue to place the responsibility for care of disabled family members on women. On the positive side, provision of paid services proposed under a revised plan for the severely disabled may allow women and other family caregivers to participate increasingly in supervisory and coordinating functions instead of providing direct personal care services.

These examples of changing families raise questions about a long-term care system that may rely heavily on home and community-based care. Families with fewer members may be closer knit and retain strong ties, or a sense of community may emerge as single-parent families unite with other households for support. Conversely, being the sole child of a single parent with no available spouse for caregiving in either generation may create conflicts when career development and childrearing needs compete with eldercare responsibilities. This situation will add to caregiver burden and may interfere with a traditional sense of responsibility for parent care.

Vulnerable Individuals and Families. David Popenoe (1994) claims that cultural complexity and an emphasis on individualism has resulted in a weakening of the social order and the family. The prevalence of disrupted or nonintact family units and their at-risk members may conflict with an emphasis on caring for older family members. Lu Ann Aday (1993) defines some at-risk groups as: those persons "living with AIDS," the mentally ill and disabled, substance or alcohol abusers, the suicide or homicide prone, members of families in which there is abuse, the homeless, and immigrants and refugees. Such persons can represent individuals at risk for disability (Aday, 1993), or they can represent persons who are too dysfunctional to become family caregivers (Yankelovich, 1994). While it is not possible to provide an accurate count of these vulnerable individuals, some figures provide a general picture of the prevalence of dysfunction that may interfere with positive family caregiving.

In 1993, the Centers for Disease Control reported that there were over 300,000 cumulative persons diagnosed with AIDS, representing a group who will require care under a proposal for long-term care (Centers for Disease Control, 1994).

Mentally ill and disabled community prevalence rates for any Diagnostic Interview Schedule per 100 adults age 18 and over were 14.0 for men and 16.6 for women in 1990 (Rosenstein, Milazzo-Sayre, & Manderscheid, 1990). While these nationally standardized figures do not represent an accurate picture of the chronically ill, they provide some picture of the numbers of chronically mentally ill and disabled family members who may not be able to care for other family members.

Depressed or suicide-prone persons represent those who are experiencing feelings of personal unfulfillment, a side-effect of an emphasis on individualism (Popenoe, 1994). Rates in 1989 for older white males 75 to 84 years of age were 55.3/100,000, and 71.9/100,000 for white males 85 years and older–these rates were much higher, for example, than those of white males age 15 to 24 years (23.2/100,000) the same year. Rates for women and persons of other races are much lower than for white men (Aday, 1993).

Families with a member who abuses alcohol may also represent a limitation in available informal caregiver resources. While prevalence rates are not available, mortality rates from 1986 to 1988 show the extent of abuse. During the high caregiving years, alcohol-related mortality rates increase, from 2.3/100,000 for ages 25 to 34 to 20.5/100,000 for ages 55 to 64. In the older years, these rates level (16.0 for 65 to 74 years; 8.9/100,000 for 75 to 84 years; and 3.2/100,000 for 85 and over) (Aday, 1993).

Physical or mental abuse is another sign of a dysfunctional family. Since women are more likely to be the recipients of abuse than men, and more likely the caregivers, this factor may add to caregiver stress in general. Elders are also recipients of abuse and neglect. Reports of abuse to women can only be estimated, but elder abuse reports for 1988 range from 2.23 to 3.96 reports per 1,000 elders although the actual prevalence is likely much higher (Tatara, 1990).

Almost seven million immigrants and refugees entered the United States between 1981 and 1989 (Aday, 1993, p. 89). They complicate the delivery of home and community-based services because of barriers in cultural practices, language, and the necessary availability of other family members. Basing social policy on a single normative national value is unrealistic. For example, in some other countries responsibility for the care of elder members is a priority (Ladd, 1976), resulting in less institutionalization than in the general U.S. population.

Family dysfunction and nontraditional family structures present an additional challenge to long-term care policy. Add to these the high rates of divorce and remarriage that compound the clear definition of responsibility for caregiving. For example, what is the responsibility of the 50-year-old woman to her relatively new 80-year-old stepfather when her mother dies? Does a family's sense of responsibility for one's parents apply in such complicated family instances? If long-term care policy can support notions of obligation, love, and responsibility in intact families, can policy positively support these feelings in the family that has become dysfunctional due to chronic physical or mental disturbances, abuse, or immigration?

Aaron and colleagues (1994) discuss social change this way: "Americans believe by overwhelming majorities that families have become weaker in ways that severely threaten human well-being and by large majorities think that weakening results from parents spending too little time with their children." Current family structures of single parents, one-parent households, or two working-parents may contribute to this trend. If so, long-term care policy with a home and community-based service emphasis cannot serve all the severely disabled without special provisions for families at risk. Whether the supports for at-risk families come through expanded governmental programs or alternative innovative models, it seems they will be needed.

Individualism. Popenoe (1994) states there is a shift since the 1950s from collective responsibility to heightened individualism resulting from economic development and cultural diversity. How this emphasis on personal goals over social or extended kinship goals will influence the duty to love and cooperate and its relationship to caregiving is unknown. Home and community-based care relies on the severely disabled having informal support and caregiving resources. On one hand, such dependency and intrafamily reliance is contrary to the heightened individualistic goals of the caregiver. The other view is that home and community-based care policy promotes individual choice and autonomy of the care recipient.

When adults responded to the question of why they provided care to elders, as in Amy Horowitz and Rose Dobrof's 1982 sample of caregivers, the reasons reported were: family responsibility, love, reciprocity, and gratitude (Doty, 1986). Suzanne Selig, Tom Tomlinson, and Tom Hickey (1991) name three reasons for caregiving: reverence, gratitude, and love. Gallup polls[3] (Gallup & Newport, 1990, 1991) reported that family life was very important to 93% of baby-boomer respondents (ages 30 to 45) and that 81% said it would become more important in the years to come (Gallup & Newport, 1990). The poll questions were too broad to know whether respondents were referring to their nuclear family or to other family members; however, Yankelovich (1994) found that Americans placed a high value on family life, with the concept of family expanded beyond the traditional nuclear form. Thus, even in an atmosphere of individualism, reaching out to help others and to care for older family members prevails.

The second view is that individuals want to retain the right to remain in their home and to make choices about their care. These expressions of individualism exemplify the priority placed on autonomy and personal choice. Proposed long-term care tax incentive policies for families in return for caregiving (Doty, 1986) are in effect a contract defining the primary caregiver and household where care will occur, eliminating choice of services and independent housing for the care recipient. When payment is made to the caregiver, such arrangements do not support individualism to the same extent that home and community-based services policy supports autonomy by reimbursing services to the disabled directly and fostering living in one's own home.

Providing expanded long-term home and community-based services may free informal caregivers for employment and other activities that exemplify individualism. Allowing for independence enhances personal and social autonomy (Clark, 1993; Popenoe, 1994). Offering reimbursement for home and community-based services may allow an increasing emphasis on individualism. In contrast, policies requiring managed care that limit individual choice of services may be incompatible with family and individual values of individualism unless the case manager develops a close trusting interpersonal relationship with the care receiver and his or her family.

DISCUSSION

The question remains: Can changing values play a part in generating family value congruence with long-term care and other health care policy proposals? Examples of federal policy provide some optimism. Recently, President Clinton signed into law the Family Leave Act providing opportunities for employees to take time from work for family responsibilities (Wisensale, 1988). Large employers like Traveler's, AT&T, and IBM have family care packages (Cowart, 1991; Stone & Kemper, 1989). Some employers establish day care centers or information and referral services to help employees with caregiving (Wisensale, 1988). As more employers support the caregiving role, family caregiving values will be further reinforced.

Other methods of supporting values related to long-term care policy have been slower to occur. Little information about values related to the care of older family members is conveyed through the secondary schools, the media, or the service networks for the disabled to provide broader education to the public and to correct misconceptions about aging and disability. Only when timing seems opportune do policy officials make a public issue of long-term care and the needs of the disabled.

One deterrent to local community influence in shaping values related to family and generational relations is that most long-term care services are in the private sector and thus are driven by market productivity. If home and other community-based care were delivered by local public or voluntary institutions such as churches, schools, or the local YMCA or YWCA, we might see a different, more diffuse impact on our sense of family and community values of collectivism. A shift from multinational corporate services to local not-for-profit agencies would reinforce use value rather than exchange value in long-term care for the disabled and elderly.

Careful analysis will be needed to determine whether restructuring long-term care policy reinforces individual and family values, that is, the utility as viewed by families regarding their own best welfare. The opposite–exchange value–as influenced by interest groups, will serve market productivity over the needs of the people. Policies that promote a balance of the two will enhance both individualism and the social order.

Yankelovich (1994) finds that major value shifts that have occurred since the 1950s include an emphasis on the ability to choose, on reciprocity rather than entitlement, and on a public desire to participate in decisions that shape people's lives. Such shifts in values may be partly due to a general fear of loss of social and individual affluence enjoyed previously (p. 19-27). Contributing to this widespread sense of uncertainty is the 1990s' atmosphere of general economic pessimism, job layoffs, forced early retirements, and an expanding service job market that has more part-time employment at lower wages and less generous private pensions and benefits plans than during the former industrial period. Despite pessimism about the future, Yankelovich (1994) emphasizes that other major values in our society such as freedom, equality before the law and of opportunity, fairness, achievement, patriotism, democracy and American exceptionalism, caring for others, and religion remain stable.

With any proposal that incorporates a heavy reliance on informal caregiving by family members, a concern for gender justice continues to nag. While values of family responsibility, love and duty are reinforced by such proposals, it is well documented that actual informal care is largely the responsibility of the female members of families. Thus, home and community-based policies are in conflict with current values that emphasize a blurring of the roles of family members related to childrearing and household responsibilities, and paid employment and career development. New policies, like the collection of current long-term policies, may drive some employed female into early retirement, placing them in financial risk for poverty in their own old age. Unfortunately, current proposals are not gender neutral, although the focus of providing an avenue of reimbursement of services without meeting a financial eligibility test may alleviate some caregiver burden and shift primary caregiver responsibility from providing direct care to coordinating and overseeing care. However, long-term care proposals emphasizing home and community-based care remain much the same as current long-term care policy in one important regard; they "reinforce(s) the nation's long-term care policy that such care is (and should remain) the responsibility of the informal sector and the unpaid labor of women" (Estes, 1991, p. 30).

As American life in the twenty-first century becomes more complex, its citizens more heterogenous, and dysfunction expands, the role of values in public policy will gain more prominence than in previous times (Popenoe, 1994). Will public policy constructively strengthen family values, or will the proposed policy create value conflicts? A different but related question is, can the current family provide the supports needed for home and community-based care without undue value conflicts? These and other related questions need further exploration, and more rigorous measures for values need to be developed.

ENDNOTES

1. Congress passed the Hill-Burton Act in 1946 to provide federal funds to support surveys, plans, and construction of new health resources including hospitals, nursing homes, and public health facilities.

2. Certificate of Need is a regulatory policy that was passed by most states in 1974 as a part of the National Health Planning and Resource Development Act. Initially passed as a way to logically distribute new hospital, nursing home, and other resources, it became a cost-containment measure and was highly politicized as firms became proficient in developing Certificate of Need justification proposals that were sold to for-profit firms. The Certificate of Need legislation is considered to be one way states rationed nursing home beds to cap Medicaid expenditures.

3. Gallup polls are conducted through 1,000 randomly selected telephone interviews with civilian noninstitutionalized adults age 18 and over.

REFERENCES

Aaron, H.J., Mann, T.E., & Taylor, T. (Eds.). (1994). *Values and public policy*. Washington, DC: The Brookings Institution.

Aday, L.A. (1993). *At risk in America: The health and health care needs of vulnerable populations in the United States*. San Francisco: Jossey-Bass Publishers.

Atchley, R.C. (1994). *Social forces and aging*, 7th edition. Belmont, CA: Wadsworth Publishing Company.

Ball, R. (1994, April). *Social security: Where are we going*? The Second Annual Pepper Distinguished Lecture, Pepper Institute on Aging and Public Policy. Tallahassee: Florida State University.

Bayles, M.D. (1987). The value of life. In D. VanDeVeer & T. Regan (Eds.), *Health care ethics: An introduction* (pp. 265-289). Philadelphia: Temple University Press.

Bengston, V. (1993). Is the "contract across generations" changing? Effects of population aging on obligations and expectations across age groups. In V.L. Bengston & W.A. Achenbaum (Eds.), *The changing contract across generations* (pp. 3-23). New York: Aldine De Gruyter.

Binstock, R.H. (1993). Older people and health care reform. *American Behavioral Scientist*, *36*(6), 823-840.

Centers for Disease Control. *Health United States 1993*. DHHS Pub. No. (PHS) 94-1232. Hyattsville, MD: National Centers for Health Statistics, U.S. Department of Health and Human Services.

Clark, P.G. (1993). Public policy in the United States and Canada: Individualism, family obligation, and collective responsibility in the care of the elderly. In J.

Hendricks & C.J. Rosenthal (Eds.), *The remainder of their days: Domestic policy and older families in the United States and Canada* (pp. 7-48). New York: Garland Publishing, Inc.

Cowart, M.E. (1991). The corporate response to caregiving. In C.N. Morrill (Ed.), *Florida caregivers handbook* (pp. 133-139). Tallahassee: Healthtrac Books.

Davis, K., Anderson, G.F., Rowland, D., & Steinberg, E.P. (1990). *Health care cost containment*. Baltimore: Johns Hopkins University Press.

Doty, P. (1986). Family care of the elderly: The role of public policy. *The Milbank Quarterly*, *64*(1), 34-75.

Doty, P. (1992). The oldest old and the use of institutional long-term care from an international perspective. In R.M. Suzman, D.P. Willis, & K.G. Manton (Eds.), *The oldest old* (pp. 251-267). New York: Oxford University Press.

Estes, C.L. (1991). The new political economy of aging: Introduction and critique. In M. Minkler & C.L. Estes (Eds.), *Perspectives on aging: The political and moral economy of growing old* (pp. 19-36). Amityville: Baywood Publishing Company, Inc.

Florida Health Care Cost Containment Board (1987). *Annual report of nursing homes*. Tallahassee: Author.

Florida Health Care Cost Containment Board (1994). *Annual report of nursing homes*. Tallahassee: Author.

Fries, J.F. (1980). Aging, natural death and the compression of morbidity. *New England Journal of Medicine*, *300*, 130-135.

Gallup, G., & Newport, F. (1990, November). Americans most thankful for peace this Thanksgiving. *The Gallup Poll Monthly*, 42-56.

Gallup, G., & Newport, F. (1991, April). Baby boomers seek more family time. *The Gallup Poll Monthly*, 31-42.

Gallup, A., & Saad, L. (1993, June). America's top health care concerns. *The Gallup Poll Monthly*, 2-5.

Garvey, E., & Logue, J.H. (1988). The community health nurse in home health and hospice care. In M. Stanhope & J. Lancaster (Eds.), *Community health nursing: Process and practice for promoting health* (pp. 805-825). St. Louis: C.V. Mosby Company.

Hareven, T.K. (1992). Family and generational relations in the later years: A historical perspective. *Generations*, *XVI*(2), 7-12.

Harrington, C., Newcomer, R.J., & Estes, C.L. (1985). *Long term care of the elderly: Public policy issues*. Beverly Hills: Sage Publications.

Hendricks, J., & Leedham, C.A. (1991). Dependency or empowerment: Toward a moral and political economy of aging. In M. Minkler & C.L. Estes (Eds.), *Critical perspectives on aging: The political and moral economy of growing old* (pp. 51-64). Amityville, NY: Baywood Publishing Company, Inc.

Kane, R.A., & Kane, R.L. (1987). *Long-term care: Principles, programs and policies*. New York: Springer Publishing Company.

Kingson, E., Hirshorn, B.A., & Cronman, J.M. (1986). *Ties that bind: The interdependence of generations*. Washington, DC: Seven Locks Press.

Ladd, J. (1976). Are science and ethics compatible? In H.T. Engelhardt & D. Callahan (Eds.), *Science, ethics and medicine* (pp. 49-78). Hastings on Hudson: The Hastings Center Institute for Society, Ethics and the Life Sciences.

Litwak, E., & Longino, C.F. (1987). Migration patterns among the elderly: A developmental perspective. *The Gerontologist, 27*, 266-272.

Longino, C.F., & Crown, W.H. (1990). Retirement migration and interstate income transfers. *The Gerontologist, 30*, 784-789.

Monk, A. (1988, December). Aging, generational continuity, and filial support. *The World & I* (a publication of the Washington Times Corporation), 549-561.

Moore, D.W. (1994, July). Public firm on health reform goals. *The Gallup Poll Monthly*, 12-18.

National Center for Health Statistics. (1994). *Advance Data No. 224. Nursing homes and board and care homes, 1991 national health provider inventory.* Hyattsville: U. S. Department of Health and Human Services.

Popenoe, D. (1994). The family condition of America: Culture change and public policy. In H.J. Aaron, T.E. Mann, & T. Taylor (Eds.), *Values and public policy* (pp. 81- 112). Washington, DC: The Brookings Institution.

Rosenstein, M.J., Milazzo-Sayre, L.J., & Manderscheid, R.W. (1990). Characteristics of persons using specialty inpatient, outpatient, and partial care programs in 1986. In R.W. Manderscheid & M.A. Sonnenschein (Eds.), *Mental health, United States, 1990* (DHHS Publication No. ADM 90-1708, pp. 139-172). Washington, DC: National Institute of Mental Health, U.S. Government Printing Office.

Selig, S., Tomlinson, T., & Hickey, T. (1991). Ethical dimensions of inter-generational reciprocity: Implications for practice. *The Gerontologist, 31*(5), 624-631.

Serow, W.J., Sly, D.F., & Wrigley, J.M. (1990). *Population aging in the United States*. New York: Greenwood Press.

Stone, R., Cafferata, G.L., & Sangl, J. (1986). *Caregivers of the elderly: A national profile*. NCHSR, Bethesda, MD: Department of HHS.

Stone, R.I., & Kemper, P. (1989). Spouses and children of disabled elders: How large a constituency for long-term care reform? *The Milbank Quarterly, 67*, 485-506.

Tatara, T. (1990). *Summaries of national elder abuse data: An exploratory study of state statistics: Based on a survey of state adult protective service and aging agencies*. Washington, DC: National Aging Resource Center on Elder Abuse.

U.S. Bureau of the Census. (1992). *1990 Census of the population: General population characteristics*. Washington, DC: U.S. Bureau of the Census.

Wiener, J.M., Illston, L.H., & Hanley, R.J. (1994). *Sharing the burden: Strategies for public and private long term care insurance*. Washington, DC: The Brookings Institution.

Wisensale, S.K. (1988). Generational equity and intergenerational policies. *The Gerontologist, 28*, 773-778.

Yankelovich, D. (1994). How changes in the economy are changing family values. In H.J. Aaron, T.E. Mann, & T. Taylor (Eds.), *Values and public policy* (pp. 16-53). Washington, DC: The Brookings Institution.

Index

